W9-BON-606

"Coughlin notes that bereavement brings about a narcissism that is nearly 'pathological.' In confessing her obsessional grief, spiralling depression and self-neglect, she wanted to reassure other bereaved people who are still setting the table for their dead husband, or waving when they see a car that looks like the deceased's, that they are not insane."

—*New York Daily News*

"What makes *Grieving* so compelling is its honest, real desperate immediacy, and the willingness of its author to struggle on the page, with her own confusion and pain without false heroism or literary posing. No one can tell you everything about grief; but Ruth Coughlin tells a great deal, and tells it beautifully, with humor, love, sorrow, frustration and hope."

—*Detroit News*

"Moving....Coughlin comes across not as a triumphant heroine but as a vulnerable human being torn by rage, confusion, and grief—one just beginning to find her way of bearing her existence."

—*Kirkus Reviews*

"Love permeates every page of Ruth Coughlin's book. I found it uplifting, and very positive. The tears I shed were for her courage, style, and honesty."

—Dominick Dunne

"A moving and touching story by an eloquent and talented writer."

—Cleveland Amory

GRIEVING

A Love Story

RUTH COUGHLIN

WITH AN INTRODUCTION BY
MICHAEL DORRIS

Harper Perennial
A Division of HarperCollins*Publishers*

Grateful acknowledgment is made to the following for permission to reprint previously published material:

Morley Music Company: Excerpt from "I'm Glad There Is You (in This World of Ordinary People)," lyrics by Paul Madeira, music by Jimmy Dorsey. Copyright © 1941, 1942 (renewed) by Morley Music Company. All rights reserved. Reprinted by permission.

A hardcover edition of this book was published in 1993 by Random House, Inc. It is here reprinted by arrangement with Random House, Inc. A short portion of this book appeared in somewhat different form in *The Detroit News.*

GRIEVING: A LOVE STORY. Copyright © 1993 by Ruth Coughlin. All rights reserved. Printed in the United States of America. No part of this book may be used or reproduced in any manner whatsoever without written permission except in the case of brief quotations embodied in critical articles and reviews. For information address Random House, Inc., 201 East 50th Street, New York, NY 10022.

HarperCollins books may be purchased for educational, business, or sales promotional use. For information, please write: Special Markets Department, HarperCollins Publishers, Inc., 10 East 53rd Street, New York, NY 10022.

First HarperPerennial edition published 1994.

Library of Congress Cataloging-in-Publication Data
Coughlin, Ruth.
    Grieving : a love story / Ruth Coughlin, with an introduction by Michael Dorris.
— 1st HarperPerennial ed.
        p.   cm.
    Previously published : New York : Random House, 1993.
    ISBN 0-06-097635-7
    I. Title.
RC265.6.C68C68   1994
155.9′37—dc20   94-10685

94 95 96 97 98 **RRD** 10 9 8 7 6 5 4 3 2 1

Introduction

Trust this book. It's true in its particulars—poignant and brave—and it's true in the wider, universal sense as well. Few of us safely escape the bitter knowledge of loss, the howling silence, the waiting and the watching, the listening, the wishing. We fight to hold on to recent memories even as, with a force like gravity, time pulls us apart from those who have died. We feel powerless, incapable of salvaging that most precious of all experiences: a normal day when we awoke without dread, without desperation, and beside the person who defines our world.

The two people you will meet and grow to care deeply about in the pages to follow are, I confide to you at the outset, as remarkable as they seem. Ruth and Bill Coughlin married in midlife and never got over their astonished gratitude in having found each other. Street smart, funny, kind, and immensely talented, they played off each other's strengths, forgave each other's failings. They could be a wisecracking pair, unsentimental in the Tracy-Hepburn mode, whose terms of endearment—"Kiddo" and "Tootsie"—were the vocabulary of equals, of a man and woman absolutely delighted at the good luck of being together. And, as you will see, they could also be, individually and as a team, heroes.

Ruth and Bill came from vastly different backgrounds, but they shared an enthusiasm for writing and were well-matched in the ability to appreciate—and to tell—a good story. They were first and ever best friends and confidants, pals, the willing straight men for each other's jokes. And oh yes: they were firmly, abidingly, and unselfconsciously in love.

I met Ruth in 1986 when, in her capacity as book editor for *The Detroit News,* she interviewed my wife, Louise Erdrich, shortly after the publication of *The Beet Queen.* Louise and I walked away from that lunch sure that we had made a friend for life. Quick, insightful, and thoroughly professional, Ruth Coughlin was someone we were anxious to know better, and the next time we were in Michigan we called to arrange a dinner with her and her husband.

Bill was a big, expansive man, hearty in every sense of the word. You knew him instantly from his eyes—intelligent, bright with good humor, careful and considerate—the kind of guy you could always count on. Highly successful both as a judge and as a writer of fiction, he was nevertheless completely unassuming, retaining the rare ability to laugh at literary pretension. The only tale I ever heard him tell twice involved the day he was a "blue-light special" while doing a book-signing at Kmart.

In the years to follow, I saw Bill in person only occasionally, but I often spoke with him on the telephone. A lifelong sufferer from asthma, he was a solid source of information and reassurance when one of our daughters was hospitalized with respiratory problems. His openhanded response was typical, for in any situation Bill was a bastion of common sense and wise perspective—savvy, perceptive, and ready to help. I know. On September 8, 1991, our oldest adopted son, Abel, the subject of my book *The Broken Cord,* was struck by a car while returning home from work and died two weeks later from his injuries. His twenty-three years of life had been marred by the permanent effects of Fetal Alcohol Syndrome, and the final senselessness of his death left Louise and me in despair. We heard from many sympathizers, friends and strangers alike, and every letter was a step on our road back to sanity. None, however, was more important or more generous than the note from Bill.

"When I die," he wrote us, "my life will have touched very few people, my immediate family and perhaps a handful of others who I have helped along the way in my professional capacity. Total, though, rather small. Abel, however, by his life, has and will affect hundreds of thousands of lives, people, probably who won't even know of his existence, but who will be healthy mentally and physically because he lived and because you recorded his life in *Broken Cord.* To live and by that life save thousands from hopeless misery isn't such a bad epitaph, I think."

How very sad, then, and yet how very appropriate, that this book, this affectionate, clear-eyed testimonial of Bill Coughlin's illness, will now touch—and instruct—thousands of readers.

vii

There's a special brand of grieving that begins with a bleak diagnosis, a terminal prognosis that inexorably, incrementally, becomes reality. Unlike the isolating, numbing blow of unexpected tragedy, anticipated death is a shared process, a delicate improvised dance of perpetual imbalance in which partners alternately hold each other up and allow each other to let go. For the person who is ill, fear of death is complicated by its practical embarrassments. For the eventual survivor, impending loss is regularly made worse by exhaustion and frustration. Yet when this pas de deux is performed with dignity and—there's no other word for it—style, no human act is braver or more ennobling. Hopeless love is love of the purest essence. It burns incandescent, brighter than any darkness, strong as a timeless star.

As a distant, periodic witness to the drama of Bill Coughlin's struggle with cancer and Ruth Coughlin's fierce, protective fight—first to beat the odds and save her husband's life and then, when that goal was clearly unattainable, to help him live his final months fully and productively—I can attest to the rightness of this book's subtitle. *Grieving* is indeed "a love story," a chronicle from which each of us will learn or be affirmed, according to our own unique experience. But of two things I feel confident: first, whether you have already faced a death, carry its enduring scars, or whether you wisely prepare yourself for the battle, Ruth Coughlin's eloquent narrative will bring courage and instill admiration in all who encounter it. And second, if Bill Coughlin read this book, he'd turn the last page, look over at Ruth, and glow with pride.

In the wholeness of life, standard happy endings are but wonderful, gracious pauses. The honesty, the day-to-day heroism of this beautifully told, unforgettable story is the genuine article, the real stuff of forever.

Michael Dorris
March 1993

Author's Note

William J. Coughlin, senior United States administrative law judge and author of fifteen novels, was my friend for fourteen years and my husband for nearly nine. On June 28, 1991, he was given a death sentence: terminal cancer. He died ten months later, on April 25, 1992, after having fought a fight akin to none other I have ever seen. He waged his battle with dignity and courage and great good faith. Without him, the sun will never be as bright.

GRIEVING

I am new to this thing called widowhood.

No one can tell you about grief, about its limitless boundaries, its unfathomable depths. No one can tell you about the crater that is created in the center of your body, the one that nothing can fill. No matter how many times you hear the word *final,* it means nothing until final is actually final.

It has been just over four months since the day Bill died, and still I am paralyzed. I am a woman without a country, an alien who has dropped to earth from some other planet. I am in a capsule on the moon, bouncing from side to side, floating in space, but I cannot imagine emerging from the capsule to offer one small step for mankind. I keep thinking I will see a 224-point headline that reads DERANGED WIDOW FOUND SUSPENDED IN OUTER SPACE, and then realize that the headline refers to me.

I rarely read newspapers, and when I do I give them only a cursory glance. Newspapers, after all, were a bond Bill and I shared, what with his reading four of them a day, and with our morning discussions about what was good in the world and what was bad in the world frequently blossoming into full-blown, morning-coffee arguments.

I have turned on the television set once—to tune in to the proceedings of the Democratic National Convention, mostly to commemorate Bill, a lifelong Democrat and a politician to his very core. At thirty-one, he had been the youngest person ever to be president of the Young Democrats, the kid who welcomed Jack Kennedy in 1960 to the state of Michigan, the same year that he himself ran for lieutenant governor. Bill would not have missed the convention for the world.

As it turned out, he did.

I am incapable of looking at baseball, the sport we both loved and watched together endlessly. I cannot remember who played in the World Series last year, and I am not inclined to find out, even though I know for a fact that we both saw every minute of it, as did we the Super Bowl.

Mail-order catalogs flood into the house, and I, a former fool and catalog maniac, throw them out immediately, not glancing at a single page. There is no piece of clothing, no trinket, no gadget I want or need.

Magazines arrive in the mail and go untouched. Because it was one of Bill's weekly rituals to do the *New York* crossword puzzle, I can barely pull the magazine out of the mailbox, let alone read it. Books, our passionate and shared interest, are tossed onto stacks in every room of the house, their spines uncracked. I will get to them someday, I know, but I cannot figure out when that day will be.

I do not play the music Bill was drawn to, from Mozart

and Mahler and Puccini to Jimmy Buffett and the Beach Boys and Nat "King" Cole. I do not turn on the radio, because I cannot decide which is worse: the thundering sound of silence that envelops me night and day or the reminder that it was Bill's habit to play the radio at all times, while he was shaving or showering or writing or reading.

There is not a second in the day that I do not long to hear his voice, listen to his advice, yearn to hear the laugh that made everyone around him smile. It is not possible for me to envision a life without him, and I know with a frightening surety that I will not be able to get along now.

I am using his toothbrush and his comb. I am wearing his shirts, their very largeness a small comfort in a universe in which comfort has been swept away. I am wearing his wedding ring, inscribed with the initials RLW, RUTH LOVES WILLIAM, on the middle finger of my left hand, right next to my own wedding ring, which I cannot contemplate ever removing.

I have taken as my own the Mont Blanc pen he so treasured, one of the last gifts I was able to give him. My old key ring has been replaced these days by the first gift I ever gave him, a gold-and-silver St. Christopher's medal suspended from a silver circle.

I have not moved his eyeglasses from the table next to our bed, and the seven dollar bills I have found in the pockets of seven of his jackets remain unspent. They never will be. I have had one of his jackets altered to fit me, sort of, in anticipation of a dark and cold winter night when I know I will prefer to wear Bill's coat rather than turn up the heat.

The Greek sailor's cap he preferred to wear once he lost his hair sits atop a pile of books in our living room. I caress it and hold it to my lips more often than I would like to admit.

In his office at home, I sit surrounded by thirty-five years of a man's life. Papers, books, letters, partial manuscripts, manuscripts that never got published, notes to himself written in his squirrelly hand—reminders of those things he hoped to accomplish on any given day. Cabinets, bursting with the accoutrements of the life that once was his, await my opening them.

In a drawer I have been able to go through for no more than a few minutes, I find his passport, one of the lottery tickets he bought every week, each bearing our special numbers—my birthday, his birthday, the date we were married—two Kennedy half-dollars, and, unaccountably, my college diploma.

If I need something from his desk, something as mundane as a paper clip, an elastic band, or one of his black felt-tip pens, I am overwhelmed by panic, opening the middle drawer so quickly and closing it so fast I know I am in danger of banging it on my fingers.

"You have to realize this is final," says Bill's doctor, with whom I have kept in touch. He is a compassionate and remarkable man, this Dr. Craig J. Gordon, this oncologist whose zeal and dedication lead him to believe that he can save the world from the corruption of cancer.

I think I know about *final* because I, who have never before seen a death certificate, now have a dozen copies of

Bill's. It is a gruesome thing, this piece of bureaucracy, this plain document stamped with its official seal, this lifeless record that has the power to destroy your sanity.

Decedent's Name: William J. Coughlin. *Informant:* Mrs. William Coughlin. *Marital Status:* Married. *Surviving Spouse* (If wife, give name before first married): Ruth Pollack. *Immediate Cause* (Final disease or condition resulting in death): Carcinoma of Unknown Primary Origin. *Cause of Death:* Abdominal carcinomatosis, Hepatic Failure related to metastatic carcinoma. *Disposition:* Cremation.

I look at this piece of paper and my vision blurs. I am underwater, I am twenty leagues beneath the sea, the air is being sucked out of my lungs, I cannot see the sky.

I have had to furnish copies of this document to too many places, too many people: the American Bar Association, the Michigan Bar Association, the lawyers for the estate, our insurance carrier, the banks behind Bill's personal credit cards, the utilities companies, the mortgage company. There are, it seems to me, far too many people who need proof that my husband is dead, and that is exactly what I have. Proof. Certification. That he is dead.

But what I am forgetting as I mail out copy after copy of this certificate is something that I did not know and am just beginning to understand.

What no one ever really tells you about is the one thing that should be the most obvious: that you will never see him again. The decedent. William J. Coughlin, deceased. He was alive one dismal, rainy Saturday afternoon in April, and then he was dead. Never to be seen again.

I know that Dr. Gordon is concerned about my welfare. I know he means to help me by discussing finality. He has, after all, seen patients die before and has been there to comfort their survivors.

"This is it," he continues. "There's no going back. You have to begin to accept it."

The idea makes the hole in the middle of my body triple in size. My heart beats faster than I can ever remember its beating before, my hands start to shake, and I begin to notice that I have forgotten how to breathe.

In these few short months since Bill's death it is difficult to know what I know or what I have learned or what lies before me. I know that I believe that life is too short. I realize it is essential to say it now, do it now, and that I must acknowledge what another Bill has told me: the secret to life is that it ends. I know it is important to cherish those things that go beyond value before you lose them, and that, as F. Scott Fitzgerald said, there are no second acts in American lives. I now agree with my mother: in life, there is no such thing as a dress rehearsal.

And as far as I can tell there is only one certainty, a certainty that is as solid as the realization that he is dead, and it is the sure knowledge that I have now learned, am continuing to learn, another language, the language of loss. Like the language of music and love, it is universal. You don't need a dictionary, you don't need a translator, you don't need a thesaurus.

8

All you need do is go through it once, just once, to get it. Bereavement. Grief. Sorrow. Mourning. Devastation. Loss. Despair. The books or newspaper articles you read or the advice you are given will or will not help you. What I have come to know is that you do what you have to do to go on. Some people will call it surviving, but you will know that it is a matter of just going on. You do what you are capable of, you do what you think will cause the least amount of pain. To yourself and to others.

There is no right or wrong to widowhood, or to loss of any kind. Nobody's written the rules, nobody can tell you how to play the game, and if they do so, the rules may or may not apply to you. You make them up as you go along.

"You must be one tough lady," a woman says when, not too long after Bill's death, I telephone Federal Express to change, for the sake of ongoing business, the account name from his name to mine. Federal Express does not require a copy of the death certificate, but this is the first time, except for having had to call the authorities, that I actually have to talk to a stranger and say that my husband is dead. I almost choke on the word, and I am embarrassed to hear the catch in my voice.

"At a time like this," the woman goes on, in a not-unkindly way, "it can't be easy. What I mean is, attending to these kinds of details, and all."

"Details and time are what I have a lot of," I respond. "The details are hard enough, what's harder is the living."

In the beginning, he said that losing his hair would not bother him.

"I'm not all that attached to my hair, you know what I mean?" Bill said, his voice, always strong, wavering almost imperceptibly on that flawlessly blue-skied day in July when we met for the first time with his oncologist, Dr. Gordon.

Oncologist. It is a word you believe you will never in your life have to use. Hear it, of course. Hear it issue from the mouths of other people, strangers, people whose suffering you can see from a distance but never have to feel. But to hear the word in connection with the one person who is your life is unthinkable, unimaginable, grotesque.

My husband's hair, then, was thick and shiny and black as night, hair I both admired and loved to touch, hair that every now and again fell with untold charm into eyes the color of the sea. The doctor, that is to say the oncologist, laughed at the line about the hair, and I laughed too, even as I tried, with little success, to imagine my husband as bald as my knee and to put into context what he was saying.

What he meant, it took me far too many minutes to understand, was that if the only thing he had to do was to sacrifice his hair in order to survive this killer called cancer, then it didn't much matter.

He had an extraordinary sense of humor, my husband did, and so for the next couple of hours he would make Dr. Craig J. Gordon laugh. About how several weeks ago when we were in Longboat Key, he couldn't understand why a wave in the Gulf of Mexico had knocked him down, rendered him breathless, and why the fall had hurt him so much.

About how the previous month, when I had taken him to another hospital because of an excruciating pain in his right side that had completely immobilized him, how that group of doctors—after having performed what seemed like every test known to the medical profession—had told us that it appeared as though there was just a small amount of fatty tissue on his liver.

About how those doctors also told us to go home and have a wonderful time.

And about how we did.

Until, that is, two weeks later when, on June 28, the biopsy report, by a bizarre twist of fate delivered by Bill's daughter Susan, a doctor herself, revealed that instead of a little fatty tissue on his liver, there was a tumor. A big one. That this large mass was malignant, that it was liver cancer, that this growth had most likely existed for a year, quietly waiting to be detected, silently preparing itself to herald Bill's death warrant.

Now, in this first exploratory meeting with Dr. Gordon, my husband was making it sound funny, even though in all the years I had known him, never once had I seen the kind of fear I saw fleetingly in his eyes now. And so we were convivial. I held my husband's hand in mine in a grip so tight I thought perhaps I was hurting him, hurting him so much that maybe a small bone might break. Because I was married to a man whose job he felt it was to cheer people up, we three would continue to laugh a great deal for the next several months. As my husband's grip on life grew weaker, my grip on his hand grew stronger. And we continued to laugh. Up to a point.

He did not in those days acknowledge that there would come a day when laughter might not be possible.

In the beginning, he said that the chemotherapy itself would not bother him.

"I'll betcha a million bucks I'll beat this," he would tell me with startling conviction. "And if I don't beat it, then at least I'll make this sucker go into remission. Hell, what's some chemotherapy if it'll buy me a few years?"

I tried, with even less success, to wonder what images were in his mind, how he was envisioning chemotherapy, nearly as horrific a word as the word *oncologist,* and how he was imagining the toll it would inevitably take.

I wondered how he could maintain such an enviable strength in mentioning, almost in passing, the fact that perhaps he might have just a few more years to live. What could it be like, I thought, for someone who had been in complete control of his life to contemplate a no-win possibility? To see, or maybe not to see, that cancer, as virulent as it sometimes can be, can spread as fast as a fire in the Hollywood hills.

Most of all, I wept and wondered about what my husband, whenever he allowed himself to do so, felt about the fact that he was dying.

Here I was thinking we would grow old together, me with those silver strands among the gold. And there he was, he with those endless reserves of optimism, goodwill, decency, and camaraderie, a man who was thinking about buying time.

He did not acknowledge then that he wouldn't be able to call the shots. He continued to say he had things to do, good works to be accomplished, a novel-in-progress to be finished, and more novels to be written. He was not ready, he said. It was not his time, he said.

In a letter to a producer in Los Angeles he wrote: "What has happened to me is very difficult to describe. I am now whipping every horse I have, hoping to see a few of them win . . . Frankly, I would have preferred to have dropped dead during the salad course. But no."

In another letter, this one to his New York literary agent, here is what he wrote, words that, until I came to know the real meaning of heartbreak, threatened to shatter my heart: "I've enjoyed several runs of luck in my life, and this may turn out to be another. We'll see."

He was playing the odds, and I was silently challenging anyone in the world to find a bookie who would bet against him.

In the beginning, he said he could hypnotize himself to the point where he could actually feel the tumor shrink. He believed in self-hypnosis, had in fact been involved in weight-loss diets that included visualization, had hypnotized colleagues and family members who wanted to stop smoking or whose fear of flying kept them on the ground.

Now he was hypnotizing himself against death.

"This is incredible," he'd say after he'd gone through the daily self-hypnosis process, smiling his special smile, the one that could light up at least a few cities.

And with the daily visualization and with the beginning jolts of the hideously powerful chemotherapy, the tumor did, unbelievably enough, shrink. I tried, with virtually no success at all, to believe, along with my husband, that it would continue to grow smaller. I had been with him—he, who never missed a trick, a guy whose powers of acuity never failed to astonish me—when we'd both listened to Dr. Gordon's prognosis.

No cure. Terminal. Only 2 percent of those stricken with cancer of the liver will survive. Four to six months, with luck, luck being the rabbit's foot my husband had apparently once carried around in the back pocket of his jeans when he was a kid. Maybe more than six months, we were told, you never know. There were cases, sure there were, where patients surprised their doctors. There were cases, sure there were, in which the chemotherapy treatments were so successful that there could be some extended time, even in the case of liver cancer.

I thought of my friend Shelby. Cancer of the liver. From

diagnosis to death, just about a week. I thought of my friend John's father. Cancer of the liver. From diagnosis to death, six weeks.

Because liver cancer rarely begins in the liver, the big search began to determine the primary site, the exact place in my husband's body where someone or some thing had decided to play a cruel joke by making crazy things happen to healthy cells.

Surgery to remove the tumor was apparently out of the question. So was a liver transplant. Same for the treatment we'd heard about that could be had only in Tokyo. And the other one, too, the one we'd been told about in Pittsburgh. There was no place we would not go, no expense we would not incur. New Zealand, no problem. Space shuttle to an unnamed planet, fine.

And so it began.

A painful operation to attempt to find the beginning of it: no dice. Other unspeakable, humiliating, and invasive tests to keep on searching. The procedure to implant what is known as a passport high up in my husband's left arm, a device that looks like a tiny button that a member of the Secret Service might use, the means through which a combination of liquid chemotherapy drugs would flow, emanating from a small black box my husband wore like a shoulder holster, a box we jokingly named Claus von Bülow, just for the hell of it.

For months, he was fine, as fine as anyone can be with a terminal illness, as fine as any man can be with a death sentence hovering like a nuclear cloud over his head. He worked, he sat on the federal bench as he had for the past seventeen years. He wrote, but never saw the publication of, his fifteenth novel. He remained relentlessly upbeat, as though nothing were wrong, dealing with people on the telephone and in person like the lifelong trouper he had already proven himself to be.

He talked a lot, as was his wont, a regular gabster he was, in that lingo that was part Raymond Chandler, part Dashiell Hammett, but always distinctly and uniquely his own.

But he rarely talked about dying. He rarely complained. Week after week after week, he thanked me for being "a real brick," he thanked me for what he called "bearing with him," three words that even now I still cannot comprehend. At least once a day he would say that he wasn't at all sure he would have the guts to take care of me the way I was taking care of him.

Guts? I would think, remembering the whimsical little coffee mug he had given me years ago, the one with the large green dragon hovering over and peering down at a small dragon-slayer clad in armor, brandishing a shield and a sword, the mug's legend reading: NO GUTS, NO GLORY. I knew exactly where the guts were in this duo. I also knew that nowhere to be seen was a scintilla of glory.

Taking care of you? I'd silently ask myself. I am watching you die and I am impotent and I want to die with you. I am watching a tornado as it spirals toward us. We are about to be drowned by the largest tsunami the world has ever witnessed, and what I really think, if you want to know the truth, is that you are taking care of me just as much as I am taking care of you.

Week after week after week, he would talk about beating it, about getting a chance to roll the dice again, about buying a boat and maybe even a summer house.

And then it got bad.

His hair, of course, was long gone, and so was the blush in his once-healthy cheeks.

He was wrong about the hair.

It turned out that the loss of it bothered him enormously, this awful, irrefutable, and visible sign that he was not a well man.

I bought baseball caps and cowboy hats by the bagful. Hat or no hat, he stopped frequenting the gas station whose customer he'd been for more than a couple of dozen years because he didn't want the guys with whom he had bantered and joked for decades to feel sorry for him. Or worse, render him, or them, speechless.

He didn't want even me to see him without a hat, which I told him was utterly silly. "I'm your wife, for God's sake," I would say. "With or without your hat, you are the handsomest man I have ever met and the one I have loved the most. Stop being ridiculous." It took me just a few times of repeating these same sentences to notice the hurt and humiliation in his eyes. To finally get it. To finally shut up. To finally know there wasn't a single, solitary thing that was ridiculous about this situation.

For our weekly visits to the oncology clinic, otherwise

known as the cancer ward, he wore that black Greek fisherman's cap he somehow managed to make look jaunty. To every nurse and every doctor who cared for him, he tipped that cap; the parking lot attendants were afforded the same small and pitiful gesture. How proud I was of him. In this simple act there was such dignity, such elegance. And, without fail, for everyone there was that thousand-watt smile, unmistakably genuine. Along with the smile, there was always a thank you.

When his temperature, inexplicably, soared beyond 103 degrees, emergency-room entrances ensued. Lots of them. The hospital stays, a week here, ten days there, were now part of the life he had left to live.

To those who had the courage to ask how he was, his answer was simple: "Not bad," he'd say, over and over again, even when it was clear that his version of "not bad" was surely something most of us would hope never in our lifetimes to encounter.

He fought.

He struggled.

He would not give up.

To those who had the courage to visit him in April—the cruelest month of all, the month he began to sleep twenty-three hours a day, the month in which he died—he would extend a frail hand, the bones now as delicate as those of a sparrow.

One of his best and longtime friends shook my husband's hand, and then opted for gallows humor. "Jesus Christ, Bill," Tom said, "at least your hands are still warm."

It worked. My husband laughed out loud. It was exactly his kind of humor.

It was exactly the kind of line Bill Coughlin would have once delivered himself and gotten exactly the laugh he was looking for.

In the end he didn't say much, but it was clear that ten months after that first diagnosis on June 28, 1991, he was not quite willing to give up.

There were, however, signs. "Kid," he said to me at one point early in April, "I think this might be it." It was a small acknowledgment that the mighty oak was about to be felled, that his immense spirit and herculean strength were soon to leave his ravaged body.

In the end, he thanked me for what he termed "all my efforts," meaning, I suppose, that he was grateful to have me around. Compared to his, my efforts were as nothing.

And at the very end, during the brutal two hours and six minutes it took for him to die in the big bed we had shared for nearly nine years, he uttered two words I had never heard him say.

"Help me," he said, almost inaudibly, but not quite.

How I wish I could have.

Not long after the diagnosis, I throw Bill a party. His fourteenth novel, *Shadow of a Doubt,* has just been published, the early reviews are raves, and I want our friends to see him still healthy, still filled with vigor, still dashing with that coal-black hair. It is, oddly, a time to celebrate, a way to pay homage to a man of many talents—lawyer, judge, novelist, and painter—who for more than twenty-five years has managed two full-time careers and is now beginning to get the recognition he has worked so long and so hard to achieve.

After all, books were how we met.

In 1978 I was working at a New York publishing house, and Bill was a judge who lived in Detroit and wrote novels. I became his editor on *The Stalking Man,* his fifth book but the first to be published in the United States, a quartet of novels having been previously published in London.

On the day of our first meeting and our first lunch, he told me that he felt very much like Herman Wouk's Youngblood Hawk. We had spent months corresponding, his letters humming with vitality and enthusiasm and a willingness to be cooperative on any editing suggestions I made. If there was a giant ego here, he was doing a good job of concealing it. We had been involved in dozens of telephone exchanges, and now it was time for us to meet face to face.

Seated across from each other at noon, I listened to him tell tales of the wild Midwest for hours. I, who had been to Chicago twice in my life and had knowledge neither of Detroit nor of the middle of America, kept thinking that in fly-over country all you did was watch the corn grow. To his eye, I must have appeared to be proof positive of the Saul Steinberg drawing in which nothing exists west of the Hudson.

More guns than people, Bill said. Place looks like the goddamned South Bronx, he said, as though he had ever set eyes on the goddamned South Bronx. Court system overloaded and gone awry, he, a former prosecuting attorney, said about what it was like to have been on the front lines in Detroit.

In his dark-blue, three-piece suit, he looked lawyerly enough, but there was a quirkiness and eccentricity to him that offset all those awful lawyer jokes. He was out to charm and impress, and I was ready to be charmed and impressed. Something told me, call it instinct, that he'd just bought the raincoat he was wearing for his big-time trip to New York, and, as it turned out, I was right.

Bill went back to Detroit late that day, in the afternoon. Many years later he confided to me that on his return flight there had been an enormous number of young children, members, in fact, of a Polish–American choir who had flown into New York to sing at a special event and who had continued to sing during the entire trip back.

A sign, he said.

When I remember the dozen long-stemmed roses, as lush and red as a cardinal's hat, that arrived at my office the next day, I think I might just have to agree with him.

And, so, thirteen years after our first meeting and not very many days after the diagnosis, of course there would be a party to celebrate Bill.

The music, you must know, is much too loud. Our best friend, Jane, who calls him Cappy, short for captain because she has always thought he should have been at the helm of a riverboat on the Mississippi, brings my husband a button for his lapel. On it is imprinted YES, I AM FAMOUS, and it makes him smile. In fact, that night he is a star; he is Clark Gable and John Wayne, he is Jimmy Cagney and Bogie all rolled into one. People form in clusters around him to hear his stories, edge nearer to his circle of light. They follow him into whichever room he moves, but mostly he stays put and holds court. The unlighted cigar, his trademark, his sole accommodation to the fact that maybe a prop is necessary to feel just a little more safe, stays firmly placed between the fingers of his right hand.

Much later, we questionably merry band form a conga line that snakes through the house, some of those in the snake's line being too young to even know what a conga line is. We revel, if you can call it that, on into the night, and there are a few of us who laugh far too much and much too boisterously.

As we clean up the usual party detritus and turn out the lights, neither Bill nor I speak. There is between us an unspoken agreement.

We will not say what we are thinking because what we are thinking is that maybe throwing a party while you are staring down the barrel of a shotgun is not such a good idea.

It is a curious thing that happens every week as I sit with Bill in the oncology clinic.

We come here for the chemotherapy to be administered, for Bill's blood to be drawn. Around us are often as many as sixty patients, here, essentially, for the same procedures.

There are people with half-faces, people with no voices, people in wheelchairs and on crutches, people with no hope. They are old and young and somewhere in between. Every once in a while a scream can be heard from one of the back cubicles, sometimes a muffled groan. It is not in the least bit unusual to hear a single sob, but the acoustics here are such that it is impossible to know where the sound is coming from.

The wait to be seen by technicians and doctors can be hours. Bill reads a newspaper, or a book, but I notice that he is not turning the book's pages at what would be his usual rapid rate. I sit both transfixed and terrified by our surroundings, expecting that Hieronymus Bosch will appear to capture this tableau. I sit and watch until I cannot bear it anymore, until there is nothing for me to do but avert my eyes.

Most of these days, I, too, bring along something to read. But here is the curious part: as soon as I open a book, I fall asleep. Straight away. Sitting up. It is like narcolepsy, but I know that I am not a narcoleptic.

What I am is a person in profound denial. What I am is someone who, in the midst of a room and a ghastly reality that would scare Stephen King, absents herself. I detest this part of me. I despise disproving what Bill appears to hold true about me, that I am made of piano wire, that I can take whatever pitch they throw at me, that I am dauntless.

Clearly, Bill is wrong.

Awakened each time by the voice of a nurse calling out the Coughlin name, I am startled, disoriented, unaware of where I am. And drowning in successive waves of guilt. How dare you? the voice inside me screams. How could you be dumb enough to doze off while your dying husband is sitting right next to you? Each time this happens, and it is rare when it does not happen, I apologize profusely and reach for his hand.

Each time, as I say I am sorry and as we gather our belongings and plow our way through the dozens of people whose suffering pulsates around us, my husband responds in precisely the same way, week after agonizing week.

"Tootsie," Bill Coughlin says, using the name we call each other at least a hundred times a day, "this has to be hard on you. You need your sleep."

When he first got sick, I bought a slew of books whose purpose was to tell me about how to cope with the presence of cancer, how to cope with my husband, how to cope with myself. A running theme throughout is the one meant to instruct me on how to prepare myself for what will happen when the victim of cancer dies.

I learned a new phrase—"anticipatory grief"—a phrase to which I devoted a great deal of thought. I considered how the experts suggest that when the situation is terminal, the person who will eventually be the cancer victim's survivor should start preparing for the finale. Intellectually. Emotionally. Literally.

The first two, I can tell you, are not possible. While Bill's fate, like Carmen's, was sealed and so, in the role of the survivor, was mine, it was beyond my ken to grasp fate's full meaning, to imagine for even one brief moment what that reality would be like.

As for the literal aspects—someone actually did question me as to why I had waited until my husband's death to make the funeral arrangements—it was hard for me to imagine how the script would be written.

Would you say to him as he lay dying, strength and hope fading like an old photograph, "Sweetheart, I'm going out for a while. Won't be long, don't worry. Just going to pick out the casket, order the thank-you cards, check with the florist, maybe get a deal if I order early"?

Many of the books enraged me, and in the main I learned little. You see the words on the page, but it is the most you can do.

If you are looking into the eye of a hurricane, there is no chance to think, to learn. What you do is run, run as fast as your feet will carry you, run like hell away from the disaster you know spells destruction.

Knowing that there was only one place to run, I became a sprinter. I ran, as I always did, to Bill. He would be my haven, he would protect me, he would keep the pain away. He would take me to safety, he would take me into the basement, as he always did when a tornado warning was in progress, and he would make sure we had enough candles in case the electricity blew. He would close the windows and draw the curtains and the shutters, as he always did, while I cowered during a thunderstorm. He would be there when I had a terrible day or when I had a good day. He would just be there.

That summer of the diagnosis was filled with balmy days. Cobalt-blue skies, opaline clouds, and night breezes soft as suede that rustled the leaves of the big old trees outside our bedroom windows.

Bill forged ahead on writing his fifteenth novel, which he titled, with a Charles Addams touch, *Death Penalty,* and I edited the pages on the computer screen and later as they came out of the printer. We continued to read much as we always did: one of us went first, the other went second, and then there was the joy of talking about the same book each of us had just finished. Sometimes, because I was a book critic, we'd have two copies of one book, and so, best of all, we would read them in tandem.

To the unknowing eye, things appeared nearly normal.

Jane and her husband, Larry, came often to visit, always filled with cheer, always telling Bill how terrific he looked. And he did. He still had his hair, he was still robust, there was still a spring to his step, and to his walk there was that familiar Bill Coughlin roll, the one that Jane was so good at imitating with perfect accuracy and enormous love after she'd run into him on a downtown street.

But Bill and I did not, for instance, acknowledge the Fourth of July. Just another holiday, we said, knowing that neither one of us could bear to think, certainly not speak out loud, that possibly this was the last Fourth of July.

We did not celebrate our wedding anniversary, nor did we exchange gifts, because on our day, July 9, we were in the hospital for Bill's laparoscopy, a procedure in which a tubular instrument is passed through a small incision in the abdominal wall to literally root around in a person's insides, to invade a person's vital organs in quest of the primary site of the cancer.

I think back to our second anniversary, the year Bill gave

me a pendant on a long gold chain, a heart fashioned from twenty-four diamonds, one for each month of our marriage, a heart I have never taken off.

"This is one helluva place for you to be on your anniversary, kiddo," Bill says to me, lying on a gurney as we wait for the surgeon to arrive. "But you know I always take you to the best places," he jokes. "First, I drag you from New York way the hell to Detroit," he goes on, "and now I'm dragging you to a hospital on your anniversary."

"It's your anniversary, too, you know," I say quietly as I lean down to kiss every part of his face, his eyes and his eyelashes, his ears, the crook of his neck, his hair, feeling a chill as I do, wondering if my husband, on our eighth wedding anniversary and eleven days after the day we learned that cancer would kill him, is already getting ready to separate himself from me.

It is the personal pronouns that give me trouble.

First person singular. First person plural. Which one am I supposed to use?

In conversation, I am accustomed to saying "our," as in, "our" garden and "our" living room. I find myself continuing to use the plural, catching myself, changing it to the singular, and then muttering, "Well, you know what I mean," to the person I am speaking to.

I note that I mention Bill's name as many times a day as possible. Retelling one of his anecdotes, referring to his thinking on an issue, pointing to his expertise and wise counsel, recounting a story that casts him in what I always see as an omniscient light, makes me feel closer to him. I imagine that this is tedious to a number of people, but I cannot stop myself.

I have taken to using phrases that are Bill's phrases, not mine. When people inquire after my welfare, I am at a loss for words. In the past, my rote response would have been, "Just fine, thanks," or sometimes, even, "Couldn't be better." Dissembling has never been one of my strong suits, but now I adopt Bill's phrase, the one he used almost up until the end: "Not bad," I now say to most who ask. My close friends don't need to ask. They know that I am close to catatonic.

I notice that Jack, Bill's much-loved, dear and loyal friend, who I often think loves Bill as much as I do, has taken to doing the same thing. Jack, an astute, savvy lawyer who knows verbal plagiarism when he sees it, does not mention that we have developed this pattern, we just do it.

Using the past tense poses a similar problem. It is like learning a new language, one I am evidently incapable of mastering. I stumble awkwardly over it, this new thing called the past tense, when I talk about Bill, embarrassing myself and, I am sure, others.

At our local bookstore, I approach the only clerk available at the counter and cannot help but notice a giant display on the shelves behind him, multiple copies of *Shadow of a Doubt* and *Death Penalty*. I am here to special order a novel the store does not currently have in stock, and in doing this, I need to give the young man my name and phone number so he'll be able to call me when the book comes in.

"Any relation?" he asks, jerking his thumb backward over his left shoulder to the shelves of books.

"Yes, he's my husband," I immediately respond, and as soon as the words are out of my mouth, I can feel the flush taking over my face. "Well, you see, what I really mean to say is that he was my husband," I go on, speaking much too fast, my hands making mechanical, jerky gestures. "See, the thing is, he died in April."

The clerk tells me he is sorry about Judge Coughlin's passing, a terminology I've never quite figured out. I mean, you're alive, then you're sick, and then you're dead, right? What is this passing business?

I am, nonetheless, touched by his offer of condolence as I feel the all-too-familiar tightness in my throat and as the tears threaten to brim over. It is November, seven months after Bill's death, and it is clear that I am not exactly on the road to recovery.

It has taken five months for me to muster the courage to sell Bill's car. While he was sick, it was on the fritz, a dead battery one week, a short in the electrical wiring another, and, throughout, our friend Scott had been generously helping me ferry it back and forth to the dealer for repairs.

The car is almost new, this huge, gleaming thing that Scott calls "the Bill boat," but now its presence, its very bigness, overwhelms me, and I know I can no longer keep it in the garage. As reminders go, a car is not something you stash handily away in a drawer. I entertain the idea of placing an ad to sell it in the paper, but the idea of anyone other than Bill test-driving it forms knots in my stomach.

I know I will take a financial loss by selling it back to the dealer, but for the moment it seems the easiest thing to do, far more easy, say, than it was going through the car to remove all of Bill's personal effects. It will be a clean sale, I expect. Drive it to the lot, contend with the used-car salesman, watch his reaction when I answer his question as to why I would be selling an almost-new car, watch him snicker ever so slightly as I accept his deal, and that will be that.

As I sit in an office waiting for him to bring me the check, I am aware that Bill's car is just where I left it on the lot, about twenty feet behind me. In the next room, I can hear another salesman making arrangements to have it driven away to be inspected, washed, cleaned, stickered. For a moment I want to stick my fingers in my ears like I did when I was six years old. I do not want to hear any of this, but I realize I should display some semblance of maturity. I will not, however, turn around when I hear one of the men turn on the Bill boat's ignition.

When the salesman reappears, he is holding something I at first do not recognize. It had never occurred to me, but now of course it does. They have to give you the license plate back, nitwit. Why didn't you even think of it?

"What am I supposed to do with this?" I ask him as he hands it over to me, license plate number FEP 885, the one I'd wave to when we often passed each other on the highway.

"You never know," he replies, "maybe someday you'll need it when you have a second car."

"Not very likely," I say. "So now that I've sold you the car, who's going to drive me home?"

The books I continue to read about being a widow seem written in Urdu, the problem, of course, being that it is impossible for me to say the word *widow*.

"There's a good piece in the *Times* today about widows," my mother tells me six weeks after Bill's death. "You should read it. It might be helpful. It's about how today widows are more independent than they used to be."

My blood surges and starts to pump, going straight to my head, setting me off balance, filling my eyes with the very redness of it. I think about how emotionally dependent I have become on Bill, and he on me, and about how this symbiosis had evolved long before he became ill. I think about how the ball has to connect with the bat only once in your life to know you've hit one out of the park and that rounding the bases to home is all that matters.

With steel in my voice, even though I know she intends well, I tell my mother I do not believe I am capable of reading this particular piece in *The New York Times* at this particular time. I mention that I don't know what to call myself these days, but *widow* is not the first thing that comes to mind.

What she doesn't know is that I, even though I think of myself as a feminist, define myself as Bill's wife. But because I am a dutiful daughter, I promise my mother that I will read the piece in the paper at some point. I place it in a drawer, where I have not yet been able to touch it.

"When do you figure you're going to get back your old personality?" an extremely dear and valued friend asks me. This is a woman, a sensitive one at that, who along with a handful of other friends has carefully watched me as I try to manage the unmanageable.

As I hear the question, it is as though a thermometer has been dropped to the floor, the mercury scattering into a thousand pieces. I watch them fly, silver and shining, as they jump randomly across the room, out of sync, out of time, out of control.

I make a stab at composure, which is not easy, inasmuch as I do not know whether to cry or to be violent or to simply get up and leave the room. I attempt to hold it in my mind that I have always believed dignity to be a virtue beyond value, and that, as Bill Coughlin's wife, nothing short of decency and kindness will do.

"Never," I say, struggling hard to think back to what my old personality was, or at least to what my old personality was perceived to be. Whatever it was, I feel as far removed from it as I do from Tokyo, where I have never been.

"Maybe someday I'll be a version of the person I once was," I tell this woman for whom I have boundless affection but now wonder if I should, "but I think I have to tell you that it is impossible to watch your husband die for ten months and then think that you will ever be the same again. Ever."

As we move into the beginning of August, Bill's optimism grows.

If Claus, the black chemotherapy box that he has described to someone as looking like a binoculars case, needs to be removed for a week because his blood counts are dangerously low—so low that if he is exposed to any sort of infection he will be dead, and not from cancer—he becomes vaguely, but only vaguely, cranky.

"This thing is a pain in the ass," he says, referring to the habits he is now compelled to learn because of this high-tech equipment. There is a whole new way of dressing, what with the long, snaking tube having to be painstakingly threaded through shirt sleeves; a whole new way of bathing, what with having to park Claus on a shelf that is already conveniently in place in the shower; a whole new sleeping position to adapt to, what with the box and its plastic case becoming a third entity in our bed.

"To tell you the whole truth," he says, using a trademark Bill Coughlin phrase, "it's the cat's ass not having to go through all this stuff, but without it, I can't help thinking that the tumor's not shrinking. If this poison isn't going into my system to kill the damn thing, then how the hell can it help but not grow?"

For a while, we transfer from the inner city oncology clinic to a suburban outpost of same, a forty-five-mile drive, one way, from our house. The suffering we see is not in any way diminished; there are simply fewer sufferers. I find myself turning into the biological mother I never was, so filled with pride and admiration to see that Bill now has an entirely new staff of nurses and fellow travelers to charm and draw near.

The reports from Dr. Gordon inform us that indeed "the thing" has become quiescent. Bill is close to exuberant, almost boyish, reminding me of a small child who has just discovered that the candy store is his.

I became his Knute Rockne, even though—because I have been involved in conversations with Dr. Gordon about which Bill knows nothing, talks that speak of the future, or, more accurately, the lack of a future—I know better. Do what you have to do, Dr. Gordon says. What we're talking about should not be considered secret. All three of us have spoken of the odds, and having been given the choice, Bill has chosen to take part in this aggressive and experimental therapy. You know your husband better than I do, says Dr. Gordon, and I can't tell you what to say or what not to say. You two decide.

What has been decided has indeed been Bill's choice. Originally, he had been told he could choose to do nothing, no treatment, no experimenting, no aggressive regimen of chemotherapy and drugs. Had he so chosen, he would have walked out of Dr. Gordon's office and known that without any treatment at all he might have four months to live, probably less.

Over time, one of the many things I have learned about my husband is that he is not a quitter. His phrases echo in my mind: "Never stop punching." "Keep your shoulder to the wheel." "Nobody but you can make it happen." "Don't leave your game in the locker room, just go out and play it." "Do the hard thing first."

Throughout our marriage, he has repeatedly told me that he wishes that if he has succeeded on any level in bringing up his six children, he hopes they have learned the one lesson he feels qualified to teach: Quit only when you know there are no other options, and at that, be doubly sure you're quitting for the right reasons.

Given the choice of giving up without a fight or entering into a pitched battle against cancer, it came as no surprise which path Bill would choose. And there was, of course, always the hope that a miracle cure would be discovered in time to save his life.

Perhaps the one thing I'd learned from the books I'd been reading was that maintaining the patient's positive attitude was paramount. Be supportive. Be understanding. Think before you speak. Be aware of the consequences of whatever you do. Choose your words carefully.

But the notion of thinking of my husband as the patient is not an easy concept to grasp.

I remember a time, years ago, when I'd dropped a tumbler in our bedroom, the slivers of broken glass covering what was then a hardwood floor, and both of us barefoot, my shoes somewhere in the room, his closer by.

"Don't dare think about moving," Bill commands, as I prepare to leap naked from our bed to tend to the dangerous situation I've just inadvertently created. "Here, put these on," he says, in a voice filled with more love than I now think I could have ever then recognized, handing me his size nine-and-a-halfs, "and then go get your own shoes and bring me back mine so I can get rid of this mess."

I remember, just two years before Bill got sick, an early morning after we'd finished having our coffee and reading the papers, with me en route back upstairs to get dressed. Halfway to the staircase, coffee cup in hand, I collapse, not knowing why, not knowing exactly when, returning to consciousness to find my nose flat against the black-and-white tiles of our foyer, a dark-blue coffee cup and a puddle of coffee at the end of my fingertips, and Bill, his face white as the underbelly of a fish, hovering over me.

A battery of tests ensued, what seemed like hundreds of them, with not a single one turning up a clue as to what had taken place that morning. There was, finally, a medical term applied to whatever it was that had happened, a term I have these days utterly forgotten, so insignificant does that term now seem and so barely worth mentioning, even if it were possible for me to dredge it up from those parts of my memory that have evidently been permanently sealed.

I do know that it was not a brain tumor; I do know that, whatever it was, it was not life-threatening.

What I know best is that when I open my eyes, after having been unconscious for however many seconds it was, I find myself cradled in my husband's arms. And then, as now, I will never forget the first thing I heard: "Jesus Christ, you scared the living hell out of me," my ultimate caretaker says to me, his voice unnaturally low. "What in the name of God do you think I would ever do if something happened to you?"

Now a something that is happening is a something whose awfulness has the terrible force of gravity, and it is happening to him. He is the patient, the sick one; I am the caretaker, the healthy one, the one who has not yet had enough schooling in how to take care.

And as far as I can tell, in what then was the early days of my limited knowledge, this is, without a doubt, a living hell—not mine, but his.

What no one ever tells you after your husband is dead is that the old chestnut about there being good days and bad days is categorically not true. There are, instead, those days that are bad, and then there are those days that are much worse. As for the nights, and very often the days, it is impossible to stop the videotape that continues to play in your mind, the months, the weeks, the last days, the last hours, the last minutes, in full color.

During the day, these days after April 25, there are things to do, a workplace, where I feel like a freak, to be reentered. More or less, I have followed the pattern that began when Bill was first diagnosed, when I would not let him see me cry because I thought it inappropriate and unseemly to show emotion in his presence, limiting uncontrollable and guilty tears to the confines of my car.

Now, as I pull into *The Detroit News* parking lot months after the day of my husband's death, I see in the rearview mirror that my good friend Michael, the poet with a camera who is otherwise known as an award-winning photographer, is pulling in directly behind me. I have been driving on the freeway for the past twenty-five minutes, brushing away hot tears from beneath my sunglasses, believing that I have gone undetected, me, this person who for more than a year has taken the act of losing it on the freeway and brought it to new heights.

It is clear that Michael has been following me all along and that we will be walking together to our mutual place of employment.

As he approaches me and my car, as I attempt to collect myself so as not to appear unseemly, I somehow manage to gather my keys and purse and book bag and swing my feet to the ground, but I know my pretense is relatively short-lived.

"Hey, darlin'," Michael greets me, his eyes telling me that, having tailed me for the entire trip downtown, he knows what he knows.

"You okay?" he asks. I can see he's trying to convince me he doesn't know what he knows.

"Never thought I'd have someone following me on the road watching me cry," I say, reaching for banter. But since my face begins to crumple like a battered envelope, banter is apparently something I've lost along the way.

Michael, throwing a comradely arm around my shoulder, tells me not to fret. He tells me that throughout his entire life, having traveled to and worked in fifty-six countries, freeways have always had the same effect on him: he just can't stop crying whenever he's on one.

I appreciate his consolation, I am grateful for his humor, and as we walk toward the *News* building, I can't stop thinking about my car, purchased in mid-August when the chemotherapy had flattened Bill to such a degree that our venturing forth to go car-shopping together was out of the question.

The car, a jazzy sort of affair, is the color of a tomato ripe enough to be picked from the vine. It is not made in America, something I know appalls Bill, who would never have considered buying a foreign-made car in his life.

But I also know that he would never impose his car rules on mine, and so I meander through dealerships not governed by the Big Three, reporting back to Bill where I stand in my thinking, seeking his advice throughout, telling him about the frequently humorous exchanges that have taken place between me and some especially strange car salespeople.

The model I ultimately choose comes in a limited number of colors, some of them simply not my style. Finally, it comes down to black or red. "What do you think?" I ask Bill. "Red, of course," he replies. "Black's too funereal."

On the night I actually drive the car of my choice off the lot, I begin to feel a sense of trepidation. Should I not have bought a Ford, a Chrysler, a Cadillac just to make Bill more comfortable?

Really, I think, would it have been such a hardship to support his native Detroit and not look like a Benedict Arnold, some non–car-driving rube from New York who doesn't have a clue about what it's like to have grown up in the city that put America on wheels?

I draw closer to our house, beginning to feel more and

more like a traitor. Not to the Big Three, for certain, but to my husband. That I am having these thoughts is peculiar to me. Before Bill became sick, my buying a new car was of little importance. In fact, in my brief driving life, I have already bought two of them.

Now, post-diagnosis, there is a heightened awareness attached to everything. It is as though each thought, each sentence, each gesture is magnified, bigger, heavier, laden with portent, freighted with a deep sense of before and after.

I press the garage-door opener, and then I see it: on the inside door leading into our house a sign has been taped. It is written in my husband's distinctive hand, this time not squirrelly in its effect.

This time, instead of a Palmer-method script that went haywire somewhere during the years of Bill's parochial-school education, the sign is crafted in big block letters on a single sheet of typing paper. It is a sign I have never removed, and it reads like this:

WELCOME SPORTS CAR DRIVERS!!

I think it was the exclamation points that did me in.

Two days after I drive my new car into the garage, Bill and I learn that my father is dead.

It is no surprise; we have been expecting this. My father has been in a nursing home for the past three years, frail of body and increasingly frail of mind. Unable any longer to care for him at home because of her own encounters with medical disaster, my mother has been visiting him and reporting to me on his health.

The week before, the week of his eighty-third birthday, my father had been moved from the nursing home to a hospital. His birthday, I imagine, was not celebrated with wild abandon in the intensive care unit where my mother tells me he is. I am sure it was a day like any other day in any other intensive care unit, a day during which monitors bleep, catheters run, and a battalion of doctors and nurses try to keep people alive. Which is what my father is. Alive. Barely.

My mother has enlisted me to call his doctors. "You'd be doing me a great favor," she tells me on the telephone from almost a thousand miles away, her voice giving way to a tiny *pop,* like a plate that's been in the oven too long. "You know how flustered I get when I talk to doctors."

All three of my father's physicians tell me in their somber voices that he is "a very sick man."

What they mean is that his lungs are filling up with fluid, that he has contracted pneumonia, that he is in congestive heart failure, that his blood pressure has dropped drastically, and that his kidneys are beginning to close down.

"Your father is amazing," the kidney specialist tells me. "Most people would be dead by now," he adds, a statement I guess is meant to elicit pride on my part but instead gives me the chills.

I know that my father for all his life has had the constitution of a Tartar crossing the steppes. I imagine him now, fragile and restrained to a bed. I know this because the treating physician tells me that it appears as though my father keeps wanting to get out, to break free from the restraints. If you were old and dying and strapped into a bed, I want to scream at this doctor, wouldn't you want to get out too?

But of course I do not.

As we receive daily reports from my mother, Bill and I discuss the inevitable. There will be no turnaround here; any day now my father's heart is going to stop beating.

"Maybe you'd better start thinking about getting ready for this," my husband advises me. I know he is not talking about my packing a suitcase or about my calling the airlines to make a reservation. "I can tell you right now, and you'd better believe it, it won't be easy."

He should know.

The year before, his own father, after whom he was named and to whom he was especially close, died at eighty-two in much the same manner. Diabetes raging out of control. A foot amputated at the ankle, a leg cut off at the knee. Congestive heart failure. Kidneys shutting down. Pneumonia, the disease Bill has always referred to as "the old man's friend." Big Bill's death brought low his only child in a way I had never before seen my husband brought low.

In talking to his father's doctors and nurses, first at the hospital and later at the nursing home, Bill had made it clear to all concerned that when the time came for his father to begin the descent, no extraordinary measures were to be taken. His father had, in fact, signed a living will. Did I agree with him? Bill asked me about his conversations with the doctors.

Yes, of course I did. By this time, Big Bill had stoically endured both amputations. A colossus, both physically and temperamentally, it was impossible to imagine him as a one-legged man for however long he was going to live. So, yes, Bill said, and I concurred: no extraordinary measures. Besides, a signed living will is a signed living will.

But when that first midnight call came to inform us that Bill's father was a few minutes away from dying, my husband, an only child, could not do it, he could not tell them to let his father go. It was the second time I had seen him cry, the first being when he told me about the death of the wife who preceded me, the mother of his six children.

"My God, he's my father," he sobbed, the words

choked, strangled, almost unintelligible, as I held him in my arms and told him there was no need to apologize for his tears. When, days later, the second call came, he knew he had to say yes.

More than a year-and-a-half later, it is clear to me that Bill remains profoundly affected by his father's death, mourns him in a quiet way, admitting, as he does, how many times during a single day that he finds his hand on the telephone, ready to dial his father's number.

"You know, I've been thinking about this a lot," Bill goes on, this time addressing the imminent death of my own father. "It's no secret he's been sick, and your mother's been in and out of hospitals for the past ten years. She's no spring chicken, either," he says, making me laugh out loud, knowing that if my mother ever heard him say this, she, a woman who thinks of herself as Tinker Bell, would be on her way to an earlier-than-expected grave.

"And what about Lucy?" Bill asks.

Lucy is my thirteen-year-old dog—in dog years, a ninety-one-year-old dowager, a mutt who in 1983 was five years old when we both made our move from New York to Michigan. And to Bill. Having confronted this Bill person and having detected that he and I now clearly comprised a matched set, Lucy is most definitely *our* dog, sleeping with us in our bed every night.

"I always figured I'd be there for you and help you when all three of them died," Bill says. "And now here I am, with this goddamned box attached to me."

He does not say anything more than that. He does not say

that even though he is wearing the goddamned box he is still dying, because at this point, just two months after the diagnosis, he will not openly admit that he is. He does not mention a word about mortality because, I have to imagine, mortality is not a concept he wants to embrace at the moment.

It is a fact, though, that the first blasts of chemotherapy have made him tired beyond knowing. They have discombobulated him, stunned him, changed him irrevocably.

"It's okay," I say. "It'll be all right. Don't you worry about it, I'll be able to handle things." I add, "And besides, who knows when anyone's going to be dying anyway?"

As I say these words, I know that I am Pinocchio. I know that my nose is growing longer by the inch. I have little certainty that I will be able to handle any of it, but it is something I will never admit.

When the telephone rings that Saturday night in August and Bill answers it, I can tell by his eyes as he talks to my mother that something is wrong. But he doesn't let on, telling me later it was his sense that this kind of news was the kind of news I should hear from my own mother, not from someone outside the family. It is apparent from this statement that he has not yet gotten it: he *is* my family.

My father is dead.

It is August 17, 1991, and we learn that he died at 7:57 P.M. I will travel the next day to New Jersey for the funeral. My brother, Michael, who lives in Los Angeles, is already there, having stopped at our parents' house on his way from London back to L.A.

There is the good dark suit that needs to be brought out from the closet and pressed, along with the good black shoes that need polishing. There is the casket to be picked out, the funeral arrangements to be made, the flowers to be bought, the discussion with the priest that has to take place.

It is impossible, of course, for Bill to come with me.

I ask Bill's son Patrick and his wife, Lynn, to stay with him in our house while I'm gone, a request at which my husband balks.

"I'm not a child, you know," he tells me with a discernible snap in his voice. "I'm a grown man, I'm perfectly capable of taking care of myself."

"I'm aware of that," I say, trying to sound neither domineering nor snarky, trying not to let on that I am unsure about what effect these poisons being pumped into my husband's body will have, trying not to let him see that I am terrified to leave him alone. What if he collapses? What if his blood counts drop? What if he needs me immediately and I am more than seven hundred miles away? There is, too, a hospital procedure that's scheduled to take place during the time I am to be gone, and under no circumstances will I let him go through this alone.

And so, Patrick and Lynn arrive. And so, I leave.

My mother and I deal with the morticians, choose the casket, buy the flowers. The line about how practice makes perfect keeps running through my mind. I wonder which set of funeral directors I will be dealing with next, the ones in New Jersey for my mother or the ones in Michigan for my husband. Or, I wonder, will I first be talking to a veterinarian? I keep thinking that it's just as well that Bill is not here, even though in his absence I am navigating without a compass. Why should he have to go through this?

My father and I have had a not-uncomplicated relationship during our life together, but he is, finally, the only father I have ever had, his blood is my blood, some of my genes are his genes, and now he is dead. A life for good or for ill has been lived, and now it is spent.

The three of us—my mother, my brother, and I—hold the wake for just one day. At eighty-three, a man doesn't have that many friends left. Bill, whom I call at least eight times a day, assures me he is fine; he sends flowers to the funeral home, as do his children, as do my friends.

It is a small band that gathers there, my aunts and uncles and cousins, my father's one surviving sister, Helen. Most of them had been to our wedding in 1983, they have met Bill, and now they know that Bill is sick and that his absence at his father-in-law's funeral is a sure sign of just how sick he is.

When they offer their condolences, they move instantly into inquiring after Bill. It isn't that they're not sad about my father, but dying at his age can hardly be seen as being picked off in your prime. Besides, going to wakes and funerals is what they've become accustomed to.

They reminisce about our wedding day, the day he told me, early in the morning, that in finding me his life had gone from black-and-white to color. They talk about how triumphant were the trumpets that sounded in the church on Park Avenue. They recall how Bill, a hambone if ever there was one, sang "Danny Boy" at the reception afterward and how blissful we looked as we danced the first dance together, he, who had once been awarded a trophy for being the Tango King of St. Clair Shores, and me, thirty-nine years old, fifteen years his junior, a not-so-blushing bride who knew just how lucky she was to be loving him.

Weddings and wakes, I think, are the only times I ever see these people.

As they ask about Bill, their eyes fill up, and their faces, to my horror, are suffused with pity.

It is hard to know who I am.

Am I a daughter at her father's funeral? Am I a wife who is about to lose her husband, a woman who just happens to be going through a dress rehearsal? I am, as it happens, both these things, but at the moment what I want to do is to stop the inexorable inevitability of the second.

I am not gone from Bill for very long; in fact, I am out of my parents' house a day earlier than scheduled. As I am getting ready to leave for the airport, Bill calls to say I should be prepared. He has taken matters into his own hands, he says. I am immediately alarmed, though I know I shouldn't be—he is alive and talking to me, isn't he?—but his voice is soothing and I sense that he is trying to turn whatever he's about to tell me into a funny story.

Just before I left for my father's funeral, Bill's hair had begun to fall out in clumps. A bunch of it on his pillow. A handful on a towel after he showered, more clumps on his shirt collar and on the shoulders of his suits. He is repulsed by this, he says, and I imagine, too, that he is frightened, what with the loss of hair being such a brutal and public acknowledgment that he is engaged in combat, recently exposed to the rigors of radiation or chemotherapy.

He just couldn't stand it anymore, he tells me now, as I feel my fingers grip the receiver and watch my knuckles turn white. He has reasoned that there was no point in waiting around for his entire head of hair to fall out, that he felt he had to take charge, be in control, demonstrate that hell, no, he just wasn't going to hang around and let it happen. Two days ago he did it, he shaved his head.

I do not know if he wept. I do not know if he attempted to put his fist through a wall. I do not know if he prayed for the strength to defeat this disease. Or if he closed his eyes for a few minutes as he ran the electric razor over his scalp. Or if, in frustration and anger displaced, he yelled at Lucy. I was not there, my absence being the first in what I will begin to see as a series of proofs displaying my many inadequacies.

"I'm just warning you," he tells me on the telephone. "I look like a big, fat toad. All I need now is a rock to sit on." He laughs. Not knowing how to respond, I laugh, too.

At the airport in Detroit, I find my brand-new car and begin to break the speed limit, pedal to the metal, fairly flying in the fast lane, racing to get home.

As I approach our house, I can see Lucy waiting for me as she always does, peering out into the dark night from the living room's floor-to-ceiling window. Through the same window, I can see Bill rise slowly from a chair as he walks to meet me at the door.

He is wearing a green-and-white Michigan State baseball cap, ever loyal to one of his alma maters. In his eyes there is expectation, shyness, shame. He is wearing a crooked and tentative smile filled with apprehension and maybe even fear.

As I curl into the envelope of his still-strong arms, I mutter into his chest that for years Yul Brynner has always turned me on, right away remembering that it was lung cancer that killed Yul Brynner.

If my husband has heard me, he does not let on. Instead, he tells me what he has told me nearly every day for as long as we have been together.

"Boy-oh-boy, Toots," he says, easing into the shortened form of our mutual term of endearment, his smile now less complicated as he buries his nose into my hair, "are you ever a sight for sore eyes."

In a desk drawer, I have personal calendars that date back to 1968. They are small leather books, not actual diaries, instead a simple accounting of what I did on any given day and with whom, archival notes spanning almost a quarter century. There have been times in my life when I have gone through these books for hours, sitting cross-legged on the floor, thinking about what a peculiar habit I have perpetuated, and also appreciating the certain continuity these shorthand records contain.

I can tell you, for instance, that on January 4, 1971, I had dinner with Ann at the Brasserie. That on April 7, 1973, my mother and I attended a performance of *Tosca* at the Met and later had dinner at the Russian Tea Room. I can tell you that, beginning February 19, 1981, Joanna and I spent a week's vacation in Sarasota, devoting a goodly amount of time to talking about how New York was a lousy place to meet a good-hearted man. And I know that on March 21, 1978, the aforementioned introductory meal with William J. Coughlin took place at La Petite Marmite, it being so attenuated a lunch that the waiters began to noisily vacuum the carpet around our feet, a not-so-subtle hint that it was time.

These days, I measure everything by two dates: June 28, 1991, the day Bill was diagnosed, and April 25, 1992, the day he died, thereby abruptly ending Calendar 1992. Since then, I have not noted a single entry, the calendar's pages remaining blank and open and lonely, eager for information, awaiting data that will prove that a life is being conducted.

Even though I have had to meet with lawyers and accountants and mortgage holders and bankers and representatives of the federal government, I cannot bring myself to mark the times or the places of these meetings. Even though I have seen friends and family and have not regretted doing so, each encounter, whether professional or personal, seems weightless. Scraps of paper scribbled with notes about where I need to be and at what hour flutter on surfaces everywhere, tossed out as soon as I return to my base of operations, which is to say, directly after I reenter the remarkably still house where my husband and I lived, the house in which he chose to die.

Because I have no permanent record, I cannot tell you the specific events that took place during the month of May. I see myself going back to work, one short week after Bill's death, believing that perhaps a modicum of solace can be found in a return to familiar routine, even though the publisher of the paper and the deputy managing editor for features both have suggested I find myself some sun and a warm beach to lie on.

It is far too soon to have gone back.

I see myself shamelessly telling people high in management, when asked how I am doing, that walking into *The Detroit News* building and resuming my job is about as meaningless and puny as anything I have ever experienced. To me, my candor seems nothing less than appropriate, but I wonder if I am committing professional suicide by being honest. Corporate is corporate is corporate, I know, and who in management wants to confront the fact that he is paying an employee who is on the floor, bleeding, almost dead, and vulnerable to being kicked? In the end, though, I reason that I have nothing left to lose, and so I continue to speak and behave honestly, which is the only thing I know how to do and maybe one of the few things I do have left.

My being on the floor and vulnerable at *The News,* however, is nothing compared to how unprotected and paranoid I am at home. Everything once familiar is now strange, unrecognizable. At every turn I expect to see Bill, and when I don't, I am shocked.

In general, I am afraid of just about everything: car-jackings, drive-by shootings, bricks and rocks being thrown from freeway overpasses, and now all my fears become untenable. I feel as though I am utterly naked all the time, and that the skin I am exposing to the whole world is thin and fragile.

These irrational feelings only intensify at home. I am frightened to be alone, each peculiar sound I hear in the night pushing me closer to a panic attack.

Even though I knew it was a necessity for a man in his

position to carry a gun, that is to say, a man who had put away hundreds of criminals, for years I fought with Bill about his being armed. I was mindful that once a madman had stormed his office and shot a security guard, but still, I hate guns, I hate people who use guns, the very sight of one makes my fingers go icy. Each night when Bill came home and I'd put my arms around him, I would often accidentally bump into it, a snub-nosed .38. Most of the time, I would laugh nervously and keep my mouth shut, knowing an argument about his having a gun wouldn't get me very far.

But every now and again I wouldn't be able to restrain myself, especially after he put the .38 in his briefcase for safekeeping. If I wanted something from the briefcase, our exchange would never vary: "Honey," he'd say, "be careful when you go in there." "Just stop telling me to be careful," I'd say. "I've got a really novel idea for you. Why don't you just get rid of the damn gun?"

Now, without Bill—and, yes, without his gun—I am exposed, insecure, my every step hesitant.

"Get a security system," my mother advises me, and for once I don't turn shirty at her suggestion, even though I tell her I feel like an idiot knowing how safe this neighborhood is. "It doesn't matter," she says, "just do it, you'll feel better."

The morning the sales representatives are scheduled to arrive, I completely forget about the appointment. The doorbell wakes me up, and, bed head and all, I charge downstairs, unprepared for them, throwing on a raincoat over my nightgown. "My God," I think to myself, "they're going to take one look at me and think I'm a bag lady."

But they are gracious and professional, and one of them already knows that I'm a widow because he has read some of Bill's books and has seen his obituary. The other young man continues to pitch me, telling me how I can save a nickel here and a dime there, and I practically cut him off midsentence. "It doesn't matter," I tell him, "this is the easiest sale you'll probably ever make in your life. Just give me whatever's the top of the line."

Two days later, it takes three men ten hours to install the top of the line, and not surprisingly, I suppose, I then become afraid to use the system. I watch the instructional video three times before I realize I'm not absorbing an iota of information about how this thing works. I know that I will inadvertently set off the alarm a number of times before I get it right, and I do.

"Maybe you should just get away for a while," a friend whose husband is out of town says, suggesting that we spend a night in Chicago. "It'll be good for you," she goes on. "You know, a change of scenery, you won't have to worry about the alarm system, we can have a nice dinner, stay in a good hotel, you can watch me shop," allowing that she understands I am not in a shopping frame of mind.

I am appreciative of her concern and support and I also think it's not such a bad idea. I am, after all, driving myself crazy at home, crying for hours at a time, and, one night, curling up into the fetal position in a corner of our bedroom and staying there far too long.

It is a good excursion, except for when my traveling companion tells me, when I suggest our going to look at a new makeup line she might like, that she thinks it's a great idea.

"Yes, let's go," she says enthusiastically. "I want you to go back to looking like my sister instead of my mother." At first I am perplexed by her comment, and then the story unfolds: earlier in the day, when we were at a different store, one of the saleswomen had referred to me as my friend's mother.

She is aghast the second she has finished the sentence. I can tell that she's mortified, and speedily I assure her not to worry, it's okay. There is a ten-year age difference between us, I being the elder, and now having been told that I apparently look at least fifteen years older than my given age, I am wounded but not entirely surprised. There are charcoal smudges beneath my eyes, my skin approximates the color of clay, the lines around my mouth have deepened, and my feet slide instead of step. I imagine that there is a penalty for death, a price you pay for letting someone die. I imagine that living alone ages you.

That night I apply the new makeup I have hastily purchased. I even buy a change of clothing. I make an effort. I pick up my feet. "You look very pretty," My Friend the Younger tells me as we leave the hotel on our way to dinner. "Thank you," I say, feeling foolish and wondering why, now that I've gone to all this trouble, I should care about how I appear to the outside world, a world that interests me not in the least. Back in Detroit, a week passes during which I continue to make an attempt at looking presentable, and then I hang it up, returning to my pre-Chicago look: damaged goods.

At home, the house becomes a memorial to Bill, with photographs of him everywhere. Since his death, I have brought out more pictures and have had them framed, have added them to the walls and to the tops of tables. The experts call it enshrinement. I call it keeping him close.

After he retired in March, Jack and Tony and Sandy and Rick have cleared out his office; they bring almost two decades' worth of boxes to the house. They bring gifts I have given him, the black ceramic bird from *The Maltese Falcon,* the stuff that dreams are made of, two enormous collages I have made for him detailing his writing career over the years. The black bird I keep upstairs in his office, which I find only fitting, along with the framed photograph of me when I was young and so was the world. I cannot bring myself to remove his robes from a carton, while the collages find a showcase spot on a downstairs wall.

"What is this," someone asks me, horror evident in her voice, "are you constructing some kind of monument here?" I am affronted by this question, even as I know how bizarre this must look to the outsider, the uninitiated; even as I know that I am turning into a modern-day Miss Havisham, the difference being, of course, that Miss Havisham was captured, frozen in time, waiting for her bridegroom on the wedding day that never took place and that I am captured, frozen in time, on the day that did take place, the day my husband died.

I find reminders everywhere.

In one of my reporter's spiral notebooks, there is a page filled with his handwriting, phone messages from the answering machine that he has jotted down. Contrary to his customary practice, he has not put a date at the top of the page, but the nature of the messages tell me they are from before June 28. It all seems from another time, a page of hieroglyphics, and of course it was from another time. It was from when Bill was breathing, when blood coursed through his veins, when his body was warm to the touch, when I could feel his hand on my back.

I do not tear out the page.

In a kitchen drawer I rarely use, I discover unopened packages of the cigars he never lighted, sticks of the sugar-free chewing gum he always preferred, in his three favorite flavors—spearmint, peppermint, bubble gum.

I leave the cigars and the gum where they are.

The closets remain filled to capacity with Bill's clothing, the bureaus brimming with socks and handkerchiefs and suspenders and gym clothes. "Oh, my," says Terri, the seamstress who has done work for both me and Bill and who now turns out to be hugely compassionate, "doesn't just the smell of him on all those shirts get to you?"

"I don't know," I respond, trying not to hurt her feelings for having raised this delicate point, "I guess I kind of find it comforting."

In saying this, I think maybe I have made a mistake; maybe what I should have done was to immediately dispose of everything, get rid of each material reminder, every evidence of who Bill was, his driver's license, his credit cards, his American Bar membership card, his blue-and-gold judge's badge.

I have, to be sure, consulted therapists. Soon after Bill was diagnosed, I returned to Fayette Loria, whom I had been seeing on and off for a while, for a couple of visits. Right after his death, there I was again. Fayette, whose only son, Josh, died when he was a young man not yet twenty, is, as always, wonderfully frank. "It never goes away," she tells me. "The pain just becomes less acute."

After Fayette, I find David R. Hough, a therapist whose specialty is bereavement counseling, especially the survivors of cancer victims. His knowledge is broad, he is comforting, he has a wry sense of humor. I tell him I think my friends and family find me tiresome, that they're becoming impatient with my inability to adjust to a life without Bill. I tell him he's the sole person I can talk to openly. "You're the only one who knows and understands," I say. "No, I'm not," he responds. "No matter what I say, you're the only one who knows."

In his practice, David has counseled hundreds of widows and widowers and survivors of loss of every stripe; he assures me that no matter how crazy I am feeling, I am not. I wonder if he is right.

In still another book I am reading about how to adjust, how to get on with my life, I note a singular piece of advice: "Remember that one is a whole number. You need not be part of a couple to enjoy yourself." I think of Shel Silverstein's *The Missing Piece* and the message it conveys: that trying to find the missing piece in order to make yourself whole can have its decided disadvantages, that you are far better off without the missing piece.

Am I the only nut case around here? I think. I found my missing piece and his name was Bill. I found myself in him and he in me and together we became one. He was my only theme. Without him, one as a whole number is pointless.

Yet another helpful hint I chance upon suggests that to get through every day and remain productive, I should make lists of things to do. I already know about lists, I've watched Bill make them for years. I am inherently not a list-maker, I am inherently a procrastinator who can diddle around for days before I actually confront the task at hand.

But, I tell myself, this could be a good idea: I'll start making lists. The advice-administering expert tells me to keep the lists short; don't expect too much of yourself, the writer cautions. My first list numbers thirty-eight items, everything from doing the laundry to buying milk to writing to Bill's publishers to replacing a button on a skirt. I am flabbergasted by this list, by its length, its very mundaneness is stupefying to me. Determined to get through it, to cross off each chore accomplished, I accomplish nothing.

The refrigerator is barren, for in the last months of his life Bill could not eat and neither could I. I figure that if I lay in a can of beer and a single orchid, I'll be a living testament to Lenny Bruce's famous line about what you're likely to find in a hooker's icebox. Food is not something that calls to me, and on those infrequent occasions when a hunger pang makes itself known, sometimes in the middle of a night without sleep, I open a tub of cottage cheese or a jar of peanut butter, only to gag after the first spoonful.

Several of my colleagues at work have commented about the weight I've lost, something I know is true because of the difference in the drape of my clothes but nothing I've verified, since I have no inclination to step on a scale. Besides, whatever loss in weight it amounts to, it does not seem that drastic to me. "You'd better start eating," one woman tells me. "Pretty soon, you'll turn sideways and we won't be able to see you."

Riding in the elevator with my friend Laura, that Brenda Starr of reporters, I wonder out loud about the instances both of us have read about people dying of heartbreak. I think of Charlie Chaplin and Oona O'Neill Chaplin, married in 1943, and the decades they were together, spending in all those years just two nights apart. If we are to believe their daughter, Geraldine Chaplin, after her father died in 1977, her mother died of heartbreak fourteen years later in 1991.

Laura shoots me a veiled glance that has become more and more familiar; filled with worry, the glance holds within it, too, a degree of alarm. She and I know that observing me is like looking at a train wreck. That morning, she has watched me go through my office, a place I have not set foot in for the past three months. She has stood by as I systematically cleaned it out, tossing reams of old and yellowing correspondence, my own clips, used notebooks, and dated memos into several trash baskets without even blinking. She has caught me staring blankly at the calendar on the wall, which is turned to the month of February, a month I cannot seem to recall.

"So, what do you think?" I ask her now in the elevator, "Is it true that people really do die of heartbreak?" I am half talking to myself, half looking for a reasoned response as I vaguely recall novels and news accounts that have addressed this phenomenon. My mind wanders as I realize, looking for logic in an illogical world, that it is not possible for a heart to break, it being, after all, muscle, not glass.

"I wonder if the heart just stops beating, or what?" I go on. "I mean, what do you figure actually happens, physiologically?"

"I don't know," Laura answers, giving the question some thought, though it's clear it is not a subject she feels like investigating right away.

"Maybe people just stop eating," she says. "Maybe they just starve to death and the cause of death is malnutrition."

We have settled into a routine. Of sorts. On the surface, it doesn't appear to vary much from our usual pattern: Bill sits on the bench, I go to work, Bill presses forward to finish *Death Penalty,* we divide the household chores, Bill sends out the mortgage payment every month, I pay the bills, we see Bill's family, we see our friends. Life as usual. Sort of.

But there are differences.

One, for instance, is that Bill, who has told me for years that reading the obituaries in *The New York Times* is for him like reading a collection of mini-novels, has stopped reading them. I can remember countless times when, constantly amazed and fascinated by the intricacy of other people's lives, he would read an especially intriguing obit aloud to me, especially one that portrayed the life of a man or woman who died at the age of, say, ninety-eight. This summer, a summer that seemed to be filled with obituaries of men in their early sixties who were victims of cancer, the same summer that Michael Landon, despite his intense public bravery, could not triumph over cancer, this part of our early-morning routine ceases to exist, its absence creating an echoing silence. It is one of the first and early signs that somewhere within Bill, hidden in a place he will not expose, at least not to me, is his acknowledgment that the days of his life will be fewer than he had counted on.

Another change is that every Tuesday we go to the clinic to see how Bill is doing, which is to say to see how, or if, the chemotherapy will be administered. There are options: will it be thrown into his body through the gas pump, as he is now given to calling the black box? Or will it be passed into his body through injection and on-the-spot intravenous infusion? The blood counts need to be checked; Dr. Gordon has advised that when Bill shaves he replace his straight-edged razor with an electric razor to guard against nicks that could literally allow him to bleed to death.

But the initial disruptive impact of the chemotherapy has abated somewhat, and the fatigue is neither as extreme nor as constant. In an eerie way, the grotesque has become the familiar.

He has taken to quoting an Irish proverb, something like: "The Devil you know is better than the Devil you don't know." It is true that we have recently been introduced to this Devil, but at the moment neither of us can bear to contemplate how devastating his final work will be.

Bill has decided that he cannot sit on the bench with a hat on his head, that the men and women who come before him have in some instances waited months and often years to appear in his court, that it is disrespectful of him to sit before them looking "stupid," in what he refers to as "a costume.'' He feels like a clown, he says, and I, shooting off my mouth in an inappropriate and unthinking manner, turn lippy and tell him that he is cuckoo. You're not getting it, I say. You're forgetting that you're the judge, you can do whatever you want, demonstrating that it is a good thing I have never been, nor will I ever be, in a position of power, so easily am I apparently inclined to abuse it.

I attempt to examine the statements I am making and decide that, in my zeal to be the coach or the cheerleader or whatever role it is that I am supposed to be trying to fill, I have gone overboard. I button my lip fast.

He decides that he wants to buy a wig, so I find what I know will be a dreadful place where we are to go. Again I speak precipitately and say we should spend however much money it takes to get a good one, a real one, one woven with real hair, both of us having observed just how bad a bad one can be. I mention a dollar figure I think we should spend, and now it is Bill's turn to snap at me. "It's temporary," he says, "there's no reason to spend that kind of money for a rug that's only going to be a stop-gap measure."

I feel the iron clamps tightening around my jaw: I know from talking to Dr. Gordon that there is no such thing as a stop-gap measure. Bill will be without hair until the day he dies. Whatever you want, it's up to you, is what I end up saying, being careful not to step over that all-too-visible line again.

The woman who sells Bill his toupee is solicitous, but not

too. She is a person who no doubt has done this a thousand times for a thousand reasons, but her manner tells me that mostly she has done it for cancer patients. We walk away with a relatively inexpensive hairpiece that tries to be the color and texture of Bill's natural hair but of course can never be.

I call Roy, who has cut Bill's and my hair for years, to tell him about the wig. He offers, without being asked, to stop by and style it, make it more individualized, more Bill-like, and we accept his offer. For an hour he snips, he trims, he shapes, chatting Bill up all the while in a manner that I can only call protective, respectful, understanding. Roy's expertise is just that, expert, but there is not a whole lot you can do with a wig that is lifeless, that has no character, that is as synthetic in its components as real life is real.

With all deference to Roy, it doesn't work. Bill thinks he looks like Howdy Doody, and worse, he says, the thing is much too hot and heavy on his head.

Quietly, very quietly, he relegates it to the top shelf of the foyer closet, where it can be seen every time we open the door for our coats. It remains there for months, a macabre symbol, with both of us pretending it doesn't exist. I toy with the idea of tossing it, but I think again. I am not in charge, it is not my wig. I am not dying, and I will not intrude. It is his decision, and if he wants it up there on the shelf, then there it will stay.

And so it is that while Bill wears a cap driving to and from the McNamara Federal Building, he takes it off when he dons his robes. The people and their lawyers, therefore, who appear before the Honorable William J. Coughlin see a man who, not by choice, has no hair on his head and who, by his choice alone, is conducting business and making decisions as though he did.

I am incapable of sleeping in our bed, the bed in which there were good times and there were bad times, the bed in which Bill died.

Two hours after his actual death, some of his children are selfless enough to change the sheets and pillowcases and sweep the nightstand's myriad pills into a carton they subsequently stash in an upstairs linen closet.

It is a moving gesture. He is, after all, their father. They, unlike me, have known him all their lives. They are now adult orphans, and I am simply the woman their father chose to take as his second wife, and yet they are thoughtful enough to help me.

They do not, however, touch the top of our dresser, which is laden with personal items, mostly Bill's—his keys, his spare change, his pen, the ten-bead rosary he always kept in his pocket, the small portable radio that was his constant companion in his last months, coexisting among my jewelry boxes and books and bottles of cologne.

Nor do they remove the framed photograph of a painting of St. Raphael that Bill's aunt, Sister Davidica, a nun who has been highly placed in the order of the Immaculate Heart of Mary all her life, had sent him during his illness.

Formerly devout but no longer a churchgoing Catholic, Bill, nonetheless, was a man of faith. When the gift arrived, I stood close to him as he read the text on the back of the photograph:

> Prayer to St. Raphael, Angel of the Sick
> May the Angel Raphael, physician in care of our health, come down from heaven to cure all who are sick and to solve the difficult problems of life . . . Be with us, O Archangel, called the Medicine of God; drive away diseases of the body and bring good health to our minds.

It was the third time I saw him cry.

"Guess old habits die hard, huh?" he said, as the tears slid from his eyes.

When Sister Davidica subsequently mailed him a medal of St. Jude, patron saint of lost causes and of the helpless, he did not cry again. Instead, he found a large safety pin, slipped the medal on it, and pinned it to a corner of the sheet on his side of the bed. "What the hell." This time he laughed. "Can't hurt, can it?"

Now I watch the dust collect and wonder when I will get around to cleaning off the dresser. Week after week, I tell Nancy, our housekeeper, not to bother with the big bedroom and Bill's office, and each time I tell her this I can see by the look on her face she thinks maybe I'm getting a little funny around the eyes. A month later, I will tell her that since there's only me, it won't be necessary for her to clean every week. Every other week will be fine, I say, and as I say it, it seems to me that she is immeasurably relieved. These days, I imagine, it can't be comfortable for an outsider to walk into a house where time has stopped.

There are those who have quietly suggested that possibly it is not such a healthy idea to stay in the house. How can you? is the line of questioning. You lived there, everything there reminds you of your life together, he died there, everything reminds you of his death there. Wouldn't it be smarter to move out, start all over again? Why don't you just sell it?

Leaving the house, I counter, would be like leaving him, and I am not yet ready to do that. I am not yet ready to erase everything we had, and besides, I say, my belligerence and hostility going into overdrive, it was natural that he die here. Moreover, I continue, do you actually imagine that I would have ever gone against his wishes? As little as we talked about his death, we did talk about the ignominy of his dying in a hospital. He and his father had been at his mother's side, in a hospital, when she died in 1972. Bill abhorred hospitals, was phobic about them. Dying in one was out of the question.

And the notion of his dying alone, all by himself in a hospital bed, is something I don't think I could ever get over. Not that I'm doing such a great job of it now.

Although I have taken it into my head that I cannot possibly sleep in our bed, I nevertheless proceed to conduct conversations with myself that go on for hours.

Don't be foolish, I say, arguing against my original decision, it's only a bed. You can do it. Toughen up. You don't need to stretch out, you can sleep on your side, just as you've been doing all these years.

It is not that I am afraid to sleep in the place where my husband breathed his final breath, fear is nowhere within me since there is no longer anything left to fear. Indeed, filled with general terror, and with the specific terror that I would be asleep when he died, I had slept next to Bill, my right arm encircling him, during the last ten months of his life, straight on through to the night before he died when he was so sick, so drugged, and so still that some people might have mistaken him for dead. No, now it is not fear, it is the dread and the darkness, the suspicion that if I climb into our bed I will never be able to climb out of it.

This dread that consumes me is equal only to the overwhelming fatigue that crushes me, grinds me down. There are days when taking a shower seems like asking too much, and there are days when for thirty minutes I stand under the nozzle's spray, losing track of time, hoping that somehow the water will diminish the despair, the aloneness, and the guilt. There are nights—and days, too—when I sleep for twelve or fourteen hours, and then there are nights when I do nothing but sit at the kitchen table and stare into the middle distance, too tired to sleep on a couch downstairs, too exhausted to drag myself upstairs into the spare room that houses another bed, the bed from my New York apartment, another bed in which Bill and I have made love.

I am distracted, disoriented, disconnected, pacing the

house in circles, mindlessly retracing my steps over and over again. Often I go out on an errand and leave without my handbag, only to discover I don't have it with me when I get to wherever it is I am going. More frequently, I do not leave the house at all unless it is an absolute necessity.

I light the unfiltered ends of filtered cigarettes and often light a cigarette while another burns steadily in an ashtray. I confuse the shampoo dispenser with the soap dispenser and find myself lathering my face with shampoo. I misplace articles of clothing, shoes, jewelry, and then spend hours trying to find them. While the telephone rings constantly, there are entire stretches of time when I turn on the answering machine and play back the messages the following day.

One afternoon I finally force myself to go looking for a new bed; it is my first and only outing toward that end, and it is an unmitigated disaster. I cannot believe I am doing this. I cannot believe I am talking to an overzealous salesman about buying a king-sized bed, which in itself sounds to me like a berserk act.

Why, after all, would I need such an enormous bed just for me? When he suggests that I test the mattress, go ahead, hop right on it, lie down and stretch my body out to judge its firmness, I, incredibly enough, do just that. Following his command like a trained circus dog, I lie on the mattress for a moment, but the tightness in my chest is such that I instantly pop right back up again. When the salesman excuses himself to go check on a possible delivery date, I uncharacteristically flee the store without waiting for him to come back.

It is apparent that I cannot seriously think about buying a new bed. I cannot think about anything except the irrefutable fact that Bill is dead. The realization, which has been strangely slow in coming to me, death certificate and all— that I will never see him again, that I will never hear his voice again, that he is extinct—hits me like a roundhouse punch. I am on the ropes and there is no one here to get me back on my feet.

At the newspaper where I work, I note that I am dividing people into two camps, those who offer their condolences and those who do not. My friend Betsy has warned me that this will happen, that she went through the same thing when her father died, but I did not think then that I would do this now.

To those who say they are sorry, I gratefully say thank you, so am I. For those who studiously avoid me, avoid looking me straight on, avoid saying a single word, I have nothing but contempt. I know that I am being small and meanspirited, I know that for many people it is difficult to approach a person locked in grief, but I know, too, that at this point in what is left of my life I am not the most forgiving person I know.

The cards and letters continue to arrive, their numbers overwhelming me, though there is no reason for me to be surprised. I keep count until I reach 136, and then I just stop counting. There are dozens of notes from people I have neither met nor heard of, people from Bill's past when he worked in the prosecutor's office and for the City of Detroit, people from the high school and colleges he attended.

There are dozens from Bill's readers, people who knew him only through his books, readers who speak of how much pleasure he has given them and who write now to say how much they will miss his novels.

"It was a shock to open the envelope and see the clip," writes Marc, who has moved from Detroit to another city and is referring to the front-page obituary written by Reed Johnson that someone has sent him, along with its photo of a beaming Bill, "and yet a smile came over my face when I saw the picture of Bill. Of course, I didn't know him well but it was always so terrific just to be around him; he was one of those rare people who always made me feel good when I saw him, whether it was at a party or dinner or even after a brief, chance encounter on the street. He was always so full of life and energy, and always seemed so happy to be alive."

I read Marc's letter a half-dozen times and then another half-dozen times, my eye focusing on two words, *alive* and *always*. Even during the bad times, Bill and I were always together, through the usual disruptions and disagreements that take place in any marriage, through sessions with a marriage counselor that proved what we already knew—that what we had was indestructible, despite the sometimes discouraging turns in his writing career or in my professional life.

Today, I think the word *always* should be stricken from the language. It is a sham, a ruse, a dirty joke, and I always knew it, too, except never as I know it now, realizing, as I must, that nothing or no one lasts forever, especially someone who was always so very happy to be alive.

"The books don't write themselves," he would say. It was one of his most-repeated lines, delivered in response to my occasional but far-too-biting harangues about our not going out enough, our being housebound because of his second career, my mewling that I was a bird trapped in a gilded cage, longing to go to a movie, to a restaurant, to a party, to go off on a vacation during which Bill was not obviously straining to come back home to write.

"If I wanted to go to the movies alone and to dinner alone, why did I even bother getting married?" I would complain. "I did all that when I was single," I'd go on, getting ready to release a ninety-mile-an-hour fastball, "and right now I'm wondering why you even bothered marrying me if all you expected me to do was hang around the house and watch you write your books."

It was a diatribe that was petulant, picayune, unfair, and absurdly simpleminded. It was, in short, egocentric, selfish, and shameless behavior. Worse, it was unconscionably fraudulent. Indeed, ours was in some ways a limited life. It was, at its most fundamental level, universal in its everydayness. No one is perfect, and certainly neither of us was; the snags that occur in all relationships surely occurred in ours. The petty grievances, the small spats, all of which now seem remarkably insignificant set against the breathtaking awareness that never again will we disagree on whether the window should be open or shut at night while we sleep.

But for all its homely elements, our life was, too, large and complex, big in its bedrock compatibility, huge in the knowledge that in the end we had each other, that our universe of two was unique to us and ours alone.

"I was so saddened to hear of Bill's death last weekend," writes Richard from Washington. "Though I didn't know him well, I have vivid memories of the gentleman at one *Detroit News* function or the other, smiling warmly and (so it seemed to me) somewhat giddily. I knew it couldn't have been the booze, since of course it was always watered down at these affairs. It took me a minute, but I did catch on—he was smiling that way because he was over-the-top in love with you. I cannot think of him now without seeing that smile. Who could blame him? Yours was, make that is, one of the great romantic stories I've ever come across . . . Thanks for showing the rest of us how."

In our almost nine years together, six of his fifteen books were published and two full manuscripts were not. The fact was, I loved editing Bill's books. I loved being a part of his writing life, being called upon, inasmuch as I had spent eighteen years in New York publishing, for my professional advice. I loved witnessing and admiring his determination and zeal as he wrote every night and both weekend days; and, yes, I loved basking in his glory, loved seeing my name on five dedication pages, so proud was I to be with him.

One year, the year before Bill got sick, because I was starting to feel alarmed by how dependent I had become on him, I went off to Paris alone. Perhaps wrongly, this dependency problem didn't bother me. Being addicted to Bill didn't seem like the worst monkey I could have on my back.

It is true that the Paris jaunt was not a pure act of independence by any means—originally I had asked Bill to come with me, but no, the book of the moment was not writing itself. My husband sent me off with good cheer, snapping a photo of me waving good-bye just before we left for the airport.

In that picture I am smiling into the camera, smiling at Bill who is grinning back at me. "You look splendid, kid," he is saying, using an adjective that time after time makes me self-conscious, but it is the adjective he chooses to bestow upon me every day. I have the last-minute jitters, stomping my childish foot and wondering out loud why I ever planned this stupid trip anyway. "Aw, c'mon," he says, "don't be silly. You just wait and see, you'll have a great time."

During the week that I am in Paris, I write three postcards a day to my husband. I am compulsive, writing to him from cafés, from restaurants, while riding buses, from the room in my hotel. I telephone him with the same frequency as I call him from my office in downtown Detroit, separated geographically from his chambers by two city blocks. When I check out of the hotel after my seven nights and six days of independence and am presented with the bill, the phone charges from Paris, France, to Grosse Pointe, Michigan, amount to $558, U.S.

Looking back now, I have no idea what I did in Paris besides write to Bill, buy him presents, and call him on the telephone. It is unclear how much money was spent on stamps.

Now, during September and October of the following year, he is determined to finish and deliver *Death Penalty* to Charles Rembar, his agent, and to HarperCollins; toward the middle of October, deliver it he does. He dispatches me to New York to meet with Cy, as he is called, to "press the flesh." Without discussing it, we both know what this means. Long before Bill was diagnosed, he informed me that he was naming me executor of his estate. Up until this point, I had known or worked with every agent and editor he had ever had, and now the message is clear: get to know the players, the ball's going to be in your court.

They were peculiar days, those days of autumn, the season to which Bill was most drawn. I see him compelled to complete the manuscript, working long hours at the computer and long after the fatigue has overtaken him.

I see Louise and Michael sending us gift after gift after gift, reminders that while they live miles away, their love and support is unflagging. One package holds rose-quartz earrings for me, another a Madonna video, just for laughs, for Bill. Handcrafted vases arrive, one so blue and perfect it takes my breath away. The following week brings a crystal apple, ruby red and dazzling, along with a six-inch round woven object that resembles a spider's web. They tell us such a thing is known among the Chippewa as a dream catcher: through its web, the bad dreams are drawn out, and through the very same web, the good dreams are caught and held. We place the dream catcher on the nightstand next to Bill's side of the bed.

I see the two of us making the ninety-mile weekly trip to the clinic, and on the good days going out afterward, Bill telling me how wonderful he feels and wouldn't it be something if he could beat it, and if not beat it entirely, maybe even see five more years. Seeing him like this, I think I actually come close to buying it, I think I actually con myself into believing that as always Bill will be right and the doctor will be wrong. I think that some small part of me believes, maybe even for just a few days, that our time will not be crazily and cruelly interrupted like a reel of film that unexpectedly snaps and breaks in the middle of the picture.

But near the end of October, there are changes; the chemotherapy is pulverizing Bill. Each day the color of his skin goes from gray to grayer, from dull to duller. One side effect of the chemotherapy is that he is losing some of his toenails, the palms of his hands are red and inflamed. And he is slowing down.

At sixty-two, his lively step of only a few months ago is turning into a sort of old man's shuffle, but I see he is trying hard not to show it. While I know there is no actual change, his broad shoulders appear to be less broad, diminished and on their way to drooping, even though he is not at this point losing weight. His eyes, once as penetrating as a laser beam, now seem veiled, as though tiny shutters have been drawn over them so that his secret thoughts will remain unseen. The long, thick black eyelashes he once trimmed regularly because they would annoyingly bat up against the lenses of his eyeglasses are becoming sparse.

Pale and short of breath, another side effect of the poisons, Bill insists on taking me to the doctor for oral surgery. Several of my teeth are infected and abscessed; they need to be pulled. The nurse has advised me that I will be put under and that I will not be able to drive myself home.

In fact, it is the oral surgeon's strict office policy that no patient arrive or leave unaccompanied. "I can call a taxi," I tell Bill, "or Jane will be more than glad to take me. I don't think you should come."

To him, this is a wholly unacceptable script.

Later, as he is folding me into bed to sleep off the aftermath of the knock-out drug, he worries if the doctor has prescribed enough pain medication. He tells me again that while he was sitting in the waiting room he has concluded that if I were really sick—and together we know what he means by this—he is certain he would not be capable of taking care of me. As I am about to drift off to a drug-induced sleep, I giggle and tell him that despite his swagger and an abundance of testosterone, he is Big Mama, the most overly protective man I have ever met in my entire life and that, hands down, he can out-nurse me in a New York minute.

Always a man with an enormous capacity to devour great quantities of food, someone who has battled the bulge all his life, Bill's appetite is now a fraction of what it once was. On our first visit to the doctor, days after the diagnosis, Bill was incredulous: "How can I have cancer?" he asked Dr. Gordon, his voice close to a plea. "From everything I've seen and read, I thought one of the first signs was an unexplained weight loss. Here I am, I'm fat and thinking everything's okay, I think I'm perfect, except that I'm fat, and now I have cancer, and look at me, I'm still fat."

Now, after decades of starvation diets, liquid diets, protein diets, low-fat diets, and regimens of hypnotism for weight loss, Bill can eat whatever he wants whenever he wants. After having eaten bushels of broccoli and cauliflower and untold pounds of broiled fish and chicken without skin, he can go hog-wild. A ton of chocolate cake, no problem. Vats of ice cream, go right ahead. Acres of pizza, pecks of French fries, and every known form of junk food, feel free.

But my husband is anything but free. He is caught in the

vise of chemotherapy, drugs with terrifying names like 5-FU and Adriamycin and Cytoxan, along with medications like Compazine and Zofran and Marinol to combat the constant nausea, these last causing Bill to drop into the deepest sleep I have ever seen him sleep almost immediately after they have been administered.

His desire for food is one of the first things to go.

In a burst of activity, I buy virtually every once-forbidden food, stocking the refrigerator and cupboards to capacity. I prepare every dish I know to be to his liking, as I did during the first months of our marriage, those days when Bill, a little sheepishly but gratified nonetheless, rapidly gained thirty-five pounds. Whole plates remain barely touched, with Bill picking at the food, pushing it around like a child who cannot bear the sight of lima beans. Quarts of ice cream begin to form freezer burn, bags of chocolate kisses stay put on the kitchen counter, their little foil skins unopened, prime cuts of beef turn that peculiar shade of gray verging on green, a sure sign of decay and rot.

Halloween, a day Bill has traditionally looked forward to with nostalgic delight because of memories past, what with him taking his six children around their neighborhood when they were "just little bitties" and because of all those leftover treats he could make disappear within minutes, goes uncelebrated.

But not unnoticed.

"No point in my going out to buy the candy this year, right?" I ask. It is, we both know, a rhetorical and not especially well-posed question. "Nah, no point," Bill answers. Our porch light off, the downstairs in darkness, Bill and I lie in bed upstairs, with Lucy between us so she won't bark at the door, waiting until we think we can no longer hear the trick-or-treaters on our street.

At about the same time, our friend Charlie tells us he is coming in from New York to do business in Detroit and will be staying overnight. He has visited us and has been our houseguest in the past, but under these changed circumstances, he is solicitous. Don't make dinner, he offers, we'll go out, I'll pay. I can stay in a hotel, don't bother. Bill will not hear of it: it is decided that I will pick Charlie up after his meeting, he will come by for drinks, we will go on to a dinner for which Bill will pick up the tab, he will stay the night with us, and I will drive him to the airport early the next morning.

We three have known each other since 1978, Charlie having met Bill at Delacorte Press the same time I did. Now a senior editor at one of Bill's publishers, he is the first person outside of friends, family, and colleagues in Detroit whom Bill has had to encounter since the diagnosis, which is to say that Charlie is the first person from Bill's New York professional life to greet him not as a life-embracing, vital force but as a man who is helplessly trapped in a riptide taking him fast from the shore he has known as his life.

Driving Charlie from his meeting to our house, I warn him not to be too shocked at Bill's appearance. I ask him if he is wary about seeing Bill, momentarily forgetting that Charlie has been in the presence of very sick people before and realizing that it is of course I who am filled with trepidation.

"Know me, know my own" has been Bill's ongoing phrase in trying to explain to me, a woman who has never experienced motherhood, certain inexplicable acts on the part of his adult children. Know me, know my own, I repeat to myself, for Bill is mine, he is my own, we are a team, and I know with certainty that this visit will be difficult for him, that he is testing himself to see how strong he will be, how in control he will appear, how hopeful he will sound.

On the surface, it is fine.

Charlie is cheerful and charming and funny and kind as he comments upon how good Bill is looking. I don't disbelieve him for a second because I understand that Charlie is expecting much worse, that he has not been with Bill every day and has not therefore seen the gradations of change over the past months.

For his part, Bill is much like the old Bill, but when Charlie and I first walk into the house, I see it: the look of embarrassment on my husband's face, the lowering of his eyes as he shakes Charlie's hand, the awful, almost-hidden acknowledgment that in his own and in Charlie's eyes he is not the man he once was and will never be again.

Our conversation is spirited, chatty, gossipy, filled with swell stories and a not-insignificant amount of laughter. And then an unexpected turn takes place.

It is the time of the ongoing William Kennedy Smith trial, about which most people in America have strong feelings, I among them, my feelings falling rather predictably on the side of Patricia Bowman and Charlie's falling in a more reasoned manner somewhere in between.

It is Bill, however, who has the strongest feelings of all. Always a man of unshakable conviction, he, the war-horse trial lawyer with years of experience in the courtroom, is now going on with great fervor about a man's being innocent until proven guilty, about the culpability of the media in convicting someone before he is tried by a jury of his peers, about what William Kennedy Smith, because of the media's reprehensible and irresponsible coverage of the case and of the trial, will have to endure for the rest of his life, even if he is proven innocent.

There is no question that Bill has always been good at arguing his point, but tonight there is a difference. Tonight he is the defense and he is arguing his case before me, the jury. Tonight there is what seems like a frenzy to his argument. Quite uncharacteristically, he is raising his voice, and with each sentence the pitch becomes louder, more strident, more impassioned. Now close to ranting, he is talking about fairness, about justice, about that statue holding those scales, about that blindfold wrapped around her eyes, about fate and the chance meeting of a young man and a young woman in a bar and the consequences of that encounter.

Sitting across the room, initially I listen to him and peer at him as though I am studying a slide beneath the lens of a microscope. Yes, I am aware that Bill is a man of passion, but here he is sounding shrill, not like himself at all. Charlie and I exchange sidelong glances; despite the fact that Charlie does not know him intimately, he knows him well enough to recognize that this behavior is un-Bill-like, a term most of our friends use when talking about Bill, even now.

As Bill continues, I see that he is directing his entire speech at me, that the fire in his eyes has once again been ignited, that I am the target of this particular brimstone.

How odd, I dumbly think to myself. He knows this whole Palm Beach thing, relative to what is going on in our lives, is not that big a deal to me. He knows that I have generally discussed it in the most superficial terms, in more of a *People* magazine style than with any real substance.

Why, I wonder, is he carrying on like this? I know my Bill, a Bill who has raised his voice at me perhaps twice. I am not put off by his behavior this night, for it is true that he has never once done anything to cause me embarrassment, whereas I run out of fingers when counting the times I have made him squirm.

Alarmed, I can't help question why, now, is he yelling at me?

Suddenly, like a sharp slap across the face, I get it.

He is furious, he is enraged, he is close to losing control because he knows that he cannot contain this disease. He is railing at the injustice of it, at his unreadiness, at his unwillingness to die, not keeling over into the salad course, as he had hoped, but helplessly standing still as he is stalked by a relentless killer. It is intolerable to him that a group of abnormal cells has collected and continues to grow, to pulse like an alien thing in a Roger Corman movie, a thing whose sole purpose is to bully him, to bring him down, to defeat him, to demonstrate in triumph how powerless he is to save his own life.

If not me, whom else would he rave at? We are indivisible, I am his other half, he is my other half, together we are one, and the third entity we have created, which has as its center Bill and me, is something I have never before known and will most likely never know again.

In railing at me, he is railing at himself. In acknowledging his impotence in the face of cancer, he recognizes, too, my utter inability to help him.

It is not William Kennedy Smith and Patricia Bowman and the media and the trial in Palm Beach.

It is my own sweet Billy, betrayed and bellowing against fate, crying out against the flickering of the flame.

The day after the funeral service, I notice that there is a small moth on a wall in the kitchen.

It is minute, perhaps equivalent to the size of my smallest finger's fingernail. It is quiescent and quite lovely to look at, pale beige, its triangular shape discernible as its little wings stay serenely flapped together. I do not see it fly, although I am aware that at various times it has moved to another part of the kitchen wall, the kitchen being the one room in the house in which I spend most of my time.

During those first paralyzing weeks after attempting to accept the unacceptable, that dead is dead is dead, that Beckett's line about the dying and the going no longer bears meaning because Bill is actually dead, I begin to fixate on this moth.

Although I do not believe in reincarnation, I convince myself this moth is Bill, despite the fact that the idea of Bill, a hulking sort of a fellow, coming back as a moth is ludicrous. I am not of the beam-me-up-Scotty school, and I have met Shirley MacLaine and believe me I am no Shirley

MacLaine, but maybe, I reason, he always wanted to be a moth.

Maybe, intensely curious and observant as he was, he always wanted to be that proverbial fly on the wall but instead has chosen to be an almost inconspicuous moth, far more elegant than a dirty and disease-carrying fly.

I do not, mind you, speak to this moth, nor do I hear this moth speaking to me, but I do take care to note his where-abouts, peaceful as he is, snoozing happily away, at least it seems to me.

I remember Styron's Peyton Loftis, recall her tragic descent into terrible madness as she imagines living inside the clock from Macy's, $39.95, and as she is haunted by the image of a flock of landbound birds who cannot fly.

Taking my wellworn copy of the book from a shelf, I page through to the passage I had marked almost thirty years ago: "I turn in the room, see them come across the tiles, dimly prancing, fluffing up their wings, I think: my poor flightless birds, have you suffered without soaring on this earth? Come then and fly. And they move on past me through the darkening sands, awkward and gentle, rustling their feathers: Come then and fly."

To know that my husband is aware that he has soared on this earth is one of the things I want to know.

To lie down in darkness is what I want to do, but for now tracking the moth is the best I can manage.

At first I tell no one about the moth, but soon I am telling anyone who will listen, noting that my moth stories are met first with silence, next with nervous laughter.

When, one morning while I am showering, I see that he is affixed to a tile high above my right shoulder, I am nonplussed that I have not seen him fly upstairs. Where had I been? What good was my vigil if not to see him take flight? And then I grin and think: Oh, Bill, you sexpot you, here you are again. I become positively sure that my husband has not left me, that he is watching over me, that he still likes to see me naked, that he has not abandoned me to try and contemplate that which is not to be contemplated, a life without him.

So this, I think, is what it's like to be on the precipice.

I think about psychics. I, an agnostic and a person who has never had faith in much of anything other than the transforming power of love, begin to imagine that someone of Bill's energy and force does not go away forever. There is some part of me that hopes there is another side, not hell, not heaven, but another side, not comprehensible to me, but just there, another side.

I hear about a trusted and well-respected psychic in the Southwest who is involved in automatic writing and can be reached by telephone and then by letter. In the letter, you are not to reveal how the person with whom you would like to be in contact died, you are only to ask three questions you want the dead person to answer, and subsequently you will be in receipt of a detailed transcript, a piece of automatic writing, in other words, Bill's answers to whatever three questions I pose.

The more I consider this, the more I am taken with the notion. I think of William Butler Yeats, whom we both admired, and his forays into automatic writing, and as I do, the more I am drawn to making contact with the psychic who will, in turn, make contact with my husband.

Surely, were I a woman of faith—say, for instance, were I a Rose Kennedy—being in touch with a psychic would never occur to me. I try to imagine Rose Kennedy and the tragedies she has endured and how she accepts God's will and does not question his decisions. I think of other people I know, surely less celebrated than Rose Kennedy, who also speak of God's will, the groups of older widows who came in force to my father-in-law's funeral, armed with their unshakable, unquestioning faith, their tranquility, working their rosary beads smooth as glass, fully accepting that God had taken his child for the better good.

I think of Frances, my mother-in-law, who has been widowed twice and who, during her first marriage, saw the death of her only child, Cathy, age six. "God has been so good to me," she tells me recently. Dumbstruck by the depth of her faith, I look at her and know at once that for her this is unequivocally true, and that I cannot connect with God the way that Frances can.

I am determined to make contact with the psychic.

But I am flummoxed: what questions will I ask? As I had fixated on the moth, I fixate now on narrowing my questions to three. The possibilities, inasmuch as Bill and I did not have numerous and lengthy discussions about his imminent death, seem boundless. The part of me that understands that my reaching the psychic is a growing obsession also understands that it is unlikely that I will ever make the call, but nonetheless I keep focusing, winnowing down the questions, sensing that if I don't obsess on something I will be close to cracking.

There is, too, another part of me that actually envisions receiving the answers to my questions, even though I know Bill's ashes and the shards of his bones are encased in a steel box in a closet behind this desk, his desk, the one at which I now sit.

These are the three I come up with:

How are you doing?

Deceptively plain in its simplicity, the answer to this one is vital to me because there were few moments in our shared life when I didn't know how he was doing, even during those times when he closed himself off and thought he was impenetrable. I need to know if he is peaceful, if he is free from pain. I need to know if he is free from the atrocities of life on earth as we know it.

Who was there to meet you at the other side?

This one is dumb, I suppose, but if I am going to get involved in this whole other-side business, this terrain to which I am loopily gravitating, I think I need to know if there was someone he loved—his mother, his father, his first wife, his best friends who died far too young, any number of women with whom he was allied long before he first married and long before he and I met.

And, last: While you were alive, did I love you enough and are you angry with me for not being able to keep you alive?

I understand this last one is off bounds because it is actually two questions posed as one, but in a mind that is careening around like a bumper car in an amusement park, I come to think that I can squeak by with this small deception.

Weeks stretch into months, and I continue to ponder these questions, my hand poised and at the ready on the telephone to make the initial call, much as my hand has been on the telephone each time I have wanted to talk to Bill, a hundred times, two hundred times, my finger punching the first three digits until I realize there is no Bill.

The questions take on a weight I delude myself into believing I can support. But the fear that my husband might actually answer these questions renders me mute.

Suppose there was no one there to meet him and he is all alone?

What if he thinks my love was inadequate, and had there been more of it, I might have saved him? The guilt seeps slowly into my body like an ink stain on a brand-new blotter.

In the end, of course, I do not make the call.

Instead I watch for my moth, hoping that the next time he decides to take flight I will be there to see the whispering flutter of his two small wings as he soars into space.

The fevers begin in early November.

Without warning, they are now suddenly part of Bill's life, soaring as they do to as high as 102 degrees, reducing his already waning strength by at least 50 percent.

He knows how to bring them down, he says; he's the father of six adult children and he remembers from when they were little: he's a pro at controlling high temperatures. While I am sure this is true, the subtext is that he does not want to go to the hospital. Since the diagnosis, he has had only one overnight stay, back in July, for the laparoscopy, and at that, he was straining to be discharged as early the next morning as possible.

I know nothing about bringing up six children and even less about high temperatures, so I am, much to Bill's annoyance, constantly on the phone with Dr. Gordon, asking for his guidance. The doctor, of course, would like me to call an ambulance for Bill and bring him to the hospital, but my husband hates ambulances even more than he hates hospitals, and who can blame him?

Even though Dr. Gordon has told us that he is always available, I feel odd about beeping him at any time of the night or day, disturbing him and his wife and his family, but I have a husband who is sick, extremely sick, and I am frantic. Whether he is stubborn is hardly the point. At the peak of a fever he begins to shake uncontrollably, and the bed linens and his pajamas become sodden, as though a rainstorm has just blown through our bedroom.

When his body shivers and his teeth chatter, I cover him with layers of blankets and quilts and lie on top of him to keep him warm. It works, but not for long.

There seems to be no explanation for these fevers, but my instructions are clear: the minute Bill's temperature reaches 103 degrees, the danger point, I am to immediately get him to the emergency room. The night that it does happen, November 23, it is fortunate that Bill's daughter Maggie, a nurse who has been traveling ten hours almost every weekend to visit her father, is staying with us.

There will be no ambulance, we will bring him there ourselves.

But there will be a hospital stay, beginning with the night when we walk Bill into the E.R. and when Dr. Gordon leaves his home to meet the three of us at midnight to tell us he is going to have to admit my husband.

As the doctor escorts Maggie and me to Maggie's car at three o'clock in the morning, as I have the sickening feeling that I have abandoned Bill in the middle of the night to the care of strangers, I put a question to Dr. Gordon.

There are ten days to this hospital stay, days in which squadrons of doctors will try to figure out what is going on, administering scores of tests. Maybe the fevers are a side effect of the chemotherapy, but no, there is nothing to indicate that the fevers and the shakes are related either to the alleged cancer-killing chemicals in his body or to the tumor that is coexisting with those same chemicals.

In a surreal turn of events, Bill tests negative for tuberculosis, but because nothing else is working, not even the intravenous antibiotics, he is put on INH therapy, drugs used for the treatment of tuberculosis.

Until this peculiar diagnosis is delivered and before Bill begins to take these medications, those who visit him in the private room where he is quarantined must wear paper masks covering the nose and mouth, doctors and nurses included, masks that dehumanize, much in the manner that Bill is dehumanized, the difference being, of course, that those of us who visit him are healthy and he is not.

On Thanksgiving Day we are alone together, my mask off as we watch the parades in New York and Hawaii and

Detroit, a lifetime tradition for Bill. In years past, I would run out on Thanksgiving morning to buy a dozen doughnuts, another lifetime tradition, and it was not unusual to see him down the whole dozen.

This year, I run out and buy six. Bill eats one.

Later in the day, we thrill at seeing the Lions heroically beat the Chicago Bears, 16–10. I watch Bill make a stab at eating an inedible slice of processed turkey smothered in canned gravy as I choke on half a bagel and a cup of cooked coffee.

We are, despite the circumstances, having a wonderful time in our narrow but wide world of two, cheering on our team, laughing at the announcers, holding hands and, in our bunker, being as close as two people can be when one of them is in a hospital bed and the other is in a chair drawn up very near to it.

I want to take a snapshot. I want to freeze this frame.

I want, most of all, to say that you can spend a whole lifetime missing the point, and that when you finally get it, it is far too late.

They have been controlled, the fevers have, at least tem-
porarily, and Bill is released on December 2, the day before
my birthday, this year a day that will be like any other day.

On December 3, I know that Bill will apologize for not
having a present for me, and I know that I will state the
obvious, that he has just been sprung from the hospital
where he has spent ten days and surely I am not expecting
a gift.

Neither am I expecting that Lucy will get sick.

Exactly thirteen years ago, the year I first met Bill, I had
paid twenty-five dollars to an animal shelter on Long Island
to purchase her, thus bestowing upon myself a thirty-fifth
birthday present. In New York in those days I had grown
tired of taking care of nothing more than a group of plants.
Thriving as they were, these plants were not showing me a
lot of heart, and heart was what I needed then, something
that Lucy, a mixture of at least two breeds, with a diamond
of white on her miraculously small breast, had a lot of. In the
car I had rented to drive Lucy and me across the bridge back
home to Manhattan, she had curled her minuscule black

body next to mine, sighed the most quiet of sighs, and rested her face just above my right knee.

Growing up, Lucy ate couches. She ate books and records and pillows and shoes, she nibbled at fine Persian rugs and felt that the legs of some very good chairs were her personal teething rings. Eventually, she grew out of it and came to be the Lucy who was there when I cried, licking the tears off my face, the Lucy who was there when I rejoiced, cavorting around, laughing with me. When louts were cruel to her, I consoled her; when they were cruel to me, her instinct was such that she curled tighter around me and smiled at me, as only dogs can smile.

Now, thirteen years later, she appears listless and slow, her eyes without luster. She looks, suddenly, much thinner than her twenty-eight pounds, and she is not bounding up and down the steps after me as I tend to my husband, who after his hospital stay is both weak and dispirited, subsisting mostly on soup and crackers, spending most of each day in bed.

"Does she seem any different to you?" I ask Bill, thinking maybe I'm just imagining this, that maybe it's true that dogs can sense when something is wrong and maybe, rather than sickness, that's what this is, her awareness that Bill is not himself.

But up until today, Lucy has seemed perfectly fine. It has been six months since Bill got sick, and during these months she has not evidenced any change. In fact, she's been perfectly fine all her life: she was a dog who was never sick. Requisite shots, yes. Sickness, no. She was a dog who never let me down, who slept in the sunshine with her front paws crossed.

She was, I thought, a dog who would never die, a dog who would be forever young, a stalwart companion who would see me through the darkest of what the bleakest days might be.

Bill admits that she does look a little sluggish, but our conversation goes no further. I am remembering the talk we had a few months ago in August, when my father was about to die. I do not know what Bill is remembering, and I am afraid to ask.

We go three times, Lucy and I do, during the next two weeks in December, to Dr. Lawrence Herzog, a blue-ribbon winner among veterinarians, whose staff is remarkable. At first, there does not appear to be great cause for alarm, and we come home, much to my and Bill's mutual relief, armed with medicines and a changed diet.

She seems to rally a bit, but two days later I bring her back to Dr. Herzog and she is hospitalized. Her heart, lungs, and kidneys are not functioning properly, and an IV unit is hooked into her beautifully turned right leg, an inelegant patch marking the place where her once-lustrous black fur had been shaved to accommodate the needle.

After four days in the hospital, I go to retrieve her, but now there is much less optimism. I sense that Dr. Herzog, who knows my husband is not well, wants to let Lucy come home one more time.

Which is what it turns out to be.

On December 17, it is clear that it is no good.

Lucy cannot eat, she is incontinent, she is barely able to move, and I need to carry her to our bedroom upstairs where she rests in her favorite spot on the foot of our bed, staring into space, close to comatose. This is a Lucy who is hanging on, but evidently proud to do even that, and Bill and I marvel at her tenacity.

"It's because she doesn't want to leave you," my husband says, as I stroke her head and her ears. As he says this, I look up at him and our eyes meet and stay met for several seconds that feel like hours. I know that he is not only talking about Lucy. I know that he means to tell me that he, too, doesn't want to leave me. And I also know that he can't say it. Not yet.

"I can't stand to see her suffer like this," I say, not knowing how else to respond.

As I bundle Lucy into my arms to take her away, it is almost impossible for me to look back at Bill. He is about to cry and so am I, but neither one of us does.

Struggling for control, I listen as he tells me how much he wishes he could come with me to Dr. Herzog's office, how I must know that what I am about to do will be difficult but that it is for Lucy's sake, that I have loved her well and long, and that it is time to put her out of her pain.

When it is over, after I have held Lucy in my arms for our last good-bye, after I have covered her poor body with kisses and have thanked her for all the years of her loyal friendship, after I have stayed away from the house long enough to gather myself together so that I can finally come back home, I walk into our bedroom and throw my coat on the low chest at the foot of our bed and lie down next to my husband.

There is nothing to say, and in the absence of speech, the tears begin. I cannot remember who is the first to weep or who is the first to comfort the other. But I do know that when I leave the bed to get another pajama top for Bill because the one he is wearing is starting to be drenched in sweat, he stops me as I am just at the door.

"Hey, Ruth?" he asks. "Would you mind doing me a favor? Do you think you could take your coat away and hang it up in the hall closet?"

At first, I do not understand.

Neither one of us has ever been a neat freak and the bedroom right now looks like Dresden after the bombing. Why all of a sudden is he asking me to hang something up?

And then I look at my coat, crunched in a heap at the bottom of our bed.

It is fur, and it is black.

There is to mourning a narcissism that borders on the pathological. At first, it is not as though you have a choice. It is not a question of whether to give in to it or not, for like an albatross with its beak pressed hard against your neck, this grief is just there. All-consuming, the desolation that hammers you can be perceived as wildly selfish and disrespectful of the world and people around you.

Someone calls to complain about his or her problems on the job, a glitch in a love affair, difficulty with a brother or sister, annoyance with the telephone company. It is true that whoever the someone is will immediately recant, apologizing for griping "at a time like this," which is invariably what the someone always says. Just as invariably, I demur, assuring the beleaguered that there is no need for apology, that life goes on, that everything is relative, and that, sure, it's both important and maddening that the cable-television repairman didn't show up when he was supposed to.

I think about what "a time like this" means, and begin to understand that what I am doing is living with the rituals of everydayness and wondering how many people I am fooling. To imply that I am oblivious to the needs of others would be neither fair nor accurate, and it is true, too, that I often think how horrible it would be to see my friends go through this. But I am acutely aware of how self-centered in this whirlpool of despair I have become. There are moments, for instance, when I would like to tell people that until you experience a loss this big, everything else is amateur night.

It is what I have come to call the dwarfing down of reality, the difference between an oak and a bonsai, the unassailable evidence that, compared to death and devastation, the rest of what passes for ordinary life is small change.

As off-track in my thinking as I may be, I try not, of course, to lash out at my friends and family; I am not that dumb. Without their love, I know that I would be in a padded room somewhere, mumbling to myself, telling my fellow inmates that I am Nefertiti or, maybe, Eleanor Roosevelt.

Instead, inanimate objects and strangers are occasionally treated to my outbursts. Rage at the computer on which I work, Bill's computer, the one that never gave him a hint of trouble and is now in the habit of regularly devouring or scrambling my work. Fury at the copying machine that keeps jamming the paper; frustrated anger at the outside front door whose latch is broken.

Ten months after April 25, 1992, junk mail addressed to Bill continues to overflow the mailbox. I know about buying and selling mailing lists and about computers spewing forth old information; I know that most of this is unavoidable, but I would like not to be opening "happy birthday" letters to Bill, printed in brightly colored ink, from life-and-accident insurance outfits.

It is the companies to whom I have, repeatedly, sent copies of the death certificate, along with detailed letters, that enrage me the most because they have not updated their information.

"Our records indicate that, even though you have a State Bar of Michigan credit card with $5,000 credit available," reads one form letter addressed to Bill from a purveyor of plastic, "if we do not hear from you by the end of next month, your credit card will expire and be closed. No replacement cards will be sent. We look forward to hearing from you. Yours sincerely."

Hell hath no fury like a widow, I say to myself, as I dial the 800 number, knowing, and not caring, that on the other end of the line will be some hapless clerk, the recipient of my wrath. I am trying to calm down as my thoughts short-circuit: What the hell do you know about expire? You think you can threaten a dead man? Go right ahead. You think you can threaten me? Just try it. Don't "yours sincerely" me with your stupid, money-grubbing solicitations. You want to know about closed, I'll tell you about closed.

I start out quietly and slowly, explaining that I have, all told, sent three successive copies of the death certificate and three accompanying letters to shut down Bill's account and that I have kept copies of my correspondence.

"We don't have any confirmation that your husband

died," the woman tells me with authority and an infuriating dose of hostility. "But don't worry about it, the account's going to be closed anyway, since we haven't heard from anybody and it's past the deadline."

I can feel my body uncoil. I am a cobra about to strike, the venom in me throbbing to be released.

"Aren't you *listening* to me?" I begin to shout. "Believe me, I'm *not* worrying about it. The account *was* closed, it's *been* closed for ten months. Do you think it's any fun for me to keep getting these letters?"

"I'm sure it isn't, ma'am," responds the woman in her best bureaucratese, using the one form of address I truly detest. "And it isn't my fault, either," she adds, an altogether unnecessary fillip.

I know it isn't, just as I know that I am sounding like a person calling from an asylum. This woman has to be wondering where I'm calling from, thinking they've locked me up and thrown away the keys, and that somehow I have escaped my cell to find a telephone booth.

"Just take his name out of the computer, okay?" I say through clenched teeth. I do not apologize, neither do I say good-bye, I simply place the receiver back in its cradle, amazed that I have managed to restrain myself from slamming down the phone.

I am ashamed of myself, and then I have an awful thought: my God, what if the woman I just hung up on is also a widow? Couldn't be, I reason. We widows understand one another, it's there in our eyes and in our voices. We are a community. We know the shame of being a widow, the person who survived, the one who couldn't save her husband, the woman who has to carry on alone but doesn't know why. Or how. A widow would never be pitiless to one of her kind.

I remember a party I attended not long ago when the hostess brought me across the room to meet another woman. "I have to introduce you two," she says, good intentions evident in her demeanor. "I just know you two have a lot in common and you'll have lots to talk about," she goes on, pausing for effect. "You're both young, recent widows." As soon as she says this, I can see she wishes she had never entertained the idea of introducing us, and my heart goes out to her. But the words are said, they have escaped her lips, and there they hang, floating in midair with nowhere to go.

For several moments this other woman and I are stunned into silence, able only to stare blankly, first at our hostess, then at each other, both of us frozen in time. There is not time to frame an answer.

Neither of us knows what to say, but somehow this painful silence has to be ended.

"How long?" I ask.

"Fourteen months," she answers. "You?"

"Nine."

We have exchanged six words, but each one is weighted with an understanding that is absolute. For the moment, there is nothing more to say; our six words and our eyes have said it all. Awkwardly we move away from each other to other parts of the house, other people, later to meet again. But for this small blip in time we have confirmed what we already know: in the fellowship of widows, shared experience is worth a thousand words.

What about resentment and bitterness? someone asks me. Aren't you furious with Bill that he died, that he abandoned you, that he left you to pick up the pieces?

Within me, I can feel something snap.

"Have you gone and lost your mind?" I ask, my voice high, squeaky, quavering, knowing that more than just a few people feel it is I who am losing my mind. "How can I be angry with him? I wasn't the one who was sick, I wasn't the one who was dying," I go on. "Nobody deserves to suffer like Bill did, except for maybe Ted Bundy, and even he didn't suffer like that. And, by the way, what are you implying? Do you think he *chose* to die and leave me?"

One night in a restaurant I see a couple seated across the room from me. They are both easily in their eighties, wrinkled as raisins, merrily downing Manhattans and smoking cigarette after cigarette after cigarette.

I cannot see what they have ordered for dinner, but I allow my imagination to picture that when their food arrives it will be a T-bone steak and a giant baked potato with butter and sour cream, and that when it comes time for dessert, each will no doubt ask for an artery-clogging confection, maybe a chocolate sundae with whipped cream and walnuts. Or maybe cheesecake.

My anger that they are alive and Bill is not is at first enormous. I cannot bring my attention back to the book I have brought along with me, but as my rage subsides somewhat I remember Bill's description, each time we'd find ourselves, on our way to and from the Keys, in the Miami airport: "God's waiting room," he'd always say, not unkindly, as we watched middle-aged children help their parents with their walkers and their wheelchairs. There was no malice in his observation, it was more a reflection of his fear of growing feeble and helpless.

"I guess it's about time for me to take hang-gliding lessons," he'd also say, right after his father and my father died, old men suffering the indignity of old men's deaths, again a not-so-subtle nod to the fact that becoming diminished and without control were two prospects he would rather not think about.

As it happened, he became both, though he managed to hang on to his dignity. He did not have the chance to grow old.

Now, as I regard this elderly couple in the restaurant, I admonish myself severely for being resentful about them. They are, actually, quite adorable, two people who seem to be having a grand old time.

Live and let live, I silently say to myself, repeating the phrase like a mantra.

Live and let live. I suppose at least I should try.

He called me Wicket, a silly little name we picked up by sheer happenstance when we were on vacation in Hawaii in 1985.

Its origin derived from a drawing we both saw, a watercolor probably, primitive in its execution, of a stick-figure image, clearly drawn by a child, of a young boy with a jubilant smile on his face and a crude circle that represented a radiating sun in the drawing's background. "One for the Wicket," the child/artist had hand-lettered at the bottom of the picture. Neither of us knew the story behind the fanciful picture. Who, for instance, was Wicket? But we were drawn to it, and for no discernible reason other than whimsy, Bill began to call me Wicket whenever it looked as though I had triumphed in any way, large or small.

"That's one for the Wicket," he would say if I won a writing award, managed to meet an unmeetable deadline, or pulled off something as simple as getting to the cleaner's to pick up his suits before the place closed.

This month, the month of December, has a ghastly feel

to it. We had gotten through Thanksgiving just fine, but now Christmas is upon us, its looming presence hardly joyful. Bill's son Dennis had flown in from Oklahoma earlier in the month; his daughter Kathleen is arriving for the holidays from San Diego. It is the gathering of the clan, with Bill's four other children, Patrick, Maggie, Billy, and Susan, who live in Michigan, visiting more frequently than usual.

It is a bad idea, I know it from the start, but I proceed with the plan anyway, compelled by who knows what. Probably pure bad judgment. I decide that we will, as always, hold Christmas dinner at our house, though the present-giving will be scaled down, and though Bill's energy level is minimal.

By now, it is so minimal that we cannot divide the usual household chores as we have in the past. Laundry, taking out the garbage: Bill. Grocery shopping, paying the bills: Ruth. Running the dishes through the dishwasher: Shared. He is, not unexpectedly, abashed by being so helpless.

One afternoon as I am leaving for the drugstore, which, given the amount of drugs Bill is taking, has become my home away from home, I can see he is preparing to make a mini-speech.

"At this rate, you know, you're going to wear yourself out," he says. "You can't do all of this without its taking its toll." If I didn't realize how important this little speech is to him, I would laugh out loud. What's he doing talking about "taking its toll," this guy who is flat on his back, weak and getting weaker? With silent respect, I let him continue.

"So I tell you what, be kind to an old man," he says sort

of jokingly because neither of us has ever considered him to be an old man. "While you're out, buy a couple dozen sets of underwear for you and for me and some more sheets. That way, as far as the laundry's concerned, you can skip a week."

Five days before Christmas, I have rushed him to the emergency room again because the pain in his right side is hitting him like a sucker punch and it is difficult for him to breathe. It is the weekend; the weekend staff is not the most competent group of professionals we have ever met, and Bill is livid. After two days in the hospital, he says he's going AMA, a medical term new to me, but then again all these terms are new to me. AMA: he will leave the hospital against medical advice, he will not be officially discharged; in other words, he will go AWOL. I nearly have to sit on him to keep him from getting out of bed and walking out.

On the telephone on Sunday, I manage to persuade Dr. Gordon to discharge him. I promise I'll bring him back if it's necessary. "Just tell the nurse you're releasing him," I say, "because if you don't, he's so mad, I think he's going to have a stroke." Maggie and I bring him home on December 22.

Now, three days before Christmas, I am trying to make him as comfortable as possible at home. From my office downtown, I bring him a copy of Robert K. Massie's *Dreadnought: Britain, Germany, and the Coming of the Great War*, a book I know is right up his alley. He dives straight into it, but after a day I see he's put it aside.

"No good?" I ask.

"No, it's great, that's not it," he responds. "It's just too heavy."

At 1,007 pages, it is indeed a doorstopper. It has not occurred to me that the book's very weight might be a problem, that his propping it up on his chest would be too much of an effort, would sap his strength.

All our life together I have castigated Bill for dog-earing the pages of books. I, who approach books with reverence and cherish the smell and feel of a book just off press the way some people delight in the smell of a new car, would berate him constantly about this disrespectful habit. It drove me crazy, and my nagging him about it drove him just as crazy, as he pointed out starchily that I reminded him of the nuns at school who used to rap his knuckles with a ruler for the very same offense.

During an afternoon while he is sleeping, I quietly remove the book from the night table at his side of the bed and steal into the bathroom with a single-edged razor. Slowly I remove the dust jacket, and then I take the blade to the boards, cutting them from the binding at the spine, pulling them away from the glue. Carefully I cut up and divide the book's 1,007 pages into small, manageable sections.

When he wakes up, I present him with my handiwork. Breaking into a big smile, a big, prediagnosis, Bill smile, he takes my hand and kisses it.

"Now, this one," he says, "this one is really one for the Wicket."

When I am not desecrating and destroying books these two days before Christmas, I am running around like a chicken without a head, shopping, cooking, doing the usual preparing, all the while wondering just why I am doing this. But I am caught. Because Bill and I do not discuss these things, I am trying to figure out the game plan on my own. If I don't hold this Christmas party, won't it look as if I'm shutting his children out? If I do go ahead with it, won't it look too much like the last Christmas? Since he has not told me to call the whole thing off, I go ahead.

But he has allowed that he doesn't feel he has the stamina to get through the entire day, and asks would it be all right if he doesn't partake for too long in the festivities, if you can call them that.

It is a bizarre day, with the children and their various spouses and their own children gathering in bits and pieces. Bill is upstairs, mustering his strength, and I run up and down to check on his progress, helping him get dressed in his best Christmas gear: a brilliant red-and-white striped shirt, snappy black trousers, shiny black shoes I can tell he's just polished, and of course, the fisherman's cap. But his face is the color of parchment, and his blue eyes are not as deeply blue as they used to be.

Downstairs, it looks like Christmas as usual, except that no one but me is running upstairs. I hear people talking and laughing, and to me it is a cacophony, the voices echoing in my ears, reverberating, getting louder, more frenzied and disembodied. I begin to feel as if I'm in a David Lynch movie, wondering when the dwarf is next going to appear.

One of the grandchildren, at four years old a darling child, senses the air of expectancy and perhaps dread, at least among those of us who are in the living room watching the staircase, waiting to hear Bill's footsteps.

The grandchild moves to the bottom of the stairs and perches on the landing, lifting his eyes upward.

"Is this the grandpa who's dying?" he innocently pipes up, asking no one in particular.

I do not remember if anyone answered him, and more than a year later, I do not know, nor will I ever need to know, if my husband did or did not hear the question.

I cannot stand the silence.

I cannot stand the screaming in my ears or the images playing and replaying before my eyes. Bill sick, Bill getting more sick, Bill dying, Bill dead, Bill in the casket. It is the first time in my life that I can even approach understanding what veterans of war mean when they talk about flashbacks.

I am determined to find another dog. My motive, not unlike fourteen years ago, is to divert my attention away from myself, for I fear that I am drowning in self-pity. I want, too, to be able to talk to someone, to take care of someone, to make some sounds that will cut through this deafening silence.

Finding a dog should be simple enough, I think, but almost instantly the idea of it consumes me with apprehension and guilt. What if you have lost your capacity to care? Suppose you bring home a dog and it gets sick? How can you be so disloyal to Lucy? How can you be so disloyal to your husband?

Because they are *dead,* the voice inside me shrieks, that's why. Because neither your dog nor your husband is ever coming back. Because if you don't do something soon you will unravel.

While losing my mind doesn't seem like an altogether bad idea at this point, it is apparent that I must have a shred of self-preservation somewhere left within me, because I do begin looking for a dog.

Laura helps me, tracking down a two-year-old through her various connections. I call and discover that the reason the dog is being put up for adoption is that its master has died a week ago, and that the master's wife has had a stroke and is unable to look after the animal.

Somehow the circumstances do not seem right.

I keep looking, checking the classifieds every day, calling around to my veterinarian, telephoning animal shelters, checking with breeders.

After a series of phone calls, I track down a woman who breeds toy poodles and is selling what she tells me is "a real winner." Eighteen months old, housebroken and trained, sweet of nature, and very beautiful.

The woman and the dog live on a farm at least an hour away from our house, but I am game, even though I know that with my notably bad sense of direction I will no doubt get lost. I do, of course, and the trip takes me two hours instead of one.

It is indeed a bucolic setting, and as I drive up what seems like a miles-long dirt road to the house, I am filled with anticipation. This is the dog for me, I think. I am going to put her in the car and take her home and hug her for hours. I will buy her chew bones and new toys and the best dog food available. I will talk to her all the time, though at first she will not understand what I am saying. She will let me know when someone is at the door, the silence will be somewhat dispelled and maybe, just maybe, I will be able to hang on to whatever is left of my sanity.

There is no question that she is a beauty, this dog. Silver and small, she seems at first a bit shy.

"Let's take her outside," says the woman, "I think she'll be more at ease there."

Out on the lawn, the dog still appears standoffish. Odd, I think, befriending dogs is usually what I'm good at. I get down on all fours in an attempt to be doglike and less threatening to her, extending my hand in a welcoming gesture. Maybe she'll understand that I'm trying to play with her. Maybe she'll start yapping happily away and everything will be okay.

And then it happens.

She opens her tiny mouth to yap, all right, but there is no sound. There she is, her tail is now wagging with friendliness, she is prancing around as she continues to open her mouth in short little takes, just as though she were barking.

But she is not barking.

Alarmed, I look up at the breeder, my eyes wide and questioning.

"Oh, yes, I forgot to mention. She's been de-barked," the woman tells me rather nonchalantly.

I have seen this once before in my life, years ago; I was horrified then, just as I am horrified now. On the telephone, I had explained to the breeder that I was a recent widow, that I was afraid to be alone, that I desperately wanted a dog to alert me to intruders, that I wanted a companion. I have just driven two hours to get a small creature who cannot communicate.

A dog with no bark. A widow with no voice. A life with no sound.

As though fired from a cannon, I am out of that farm like a shot, racing back to my car with the speed of a champion greyhound.

On the way back, I cannot stop sobbing. I am crying for Bill, I am crying for Lucy, I am crying for this poor little dog who would like to speak but cannot. And, yes, without question, I am crying for me.

Once I get home, I resolve that I will never get attached to anyone or anything ever again. I will not hold on to anything, I will not keep anyone close.

Dependency is bad for you, I remind myself, look where it's gotten you. You are adrift at sea, there is no land in sight, and the Coast Guard has gone out of business.

That night I sleep a shallow sleep filled with fragmented dreams, most of which I do not remember. Except for the one in which Bill appears, the first time since his death that he has been present in any dream of mine other than the daily waking nightmares.

He is in our bedroom, sitting on the floor in front of the closet, which is puzzling to me since I have never in my life seen him sit on any floor, anywhere, at any time. He is, for some inexplicable reason, clutching a pillow as though to keep it close to his body, and he is looking at me with great sadness.

He does not say a word.

The next morning, a Saturday, I am newly determined. I notice that in the disaster that was Friday, I had not checked *The Detroit News* classifieds, and I do so now.

Toy poodle. Female. Eight weeks old. Black now, will turn silver. Nice disposition.

Having been told by the owner that several other people are already booked to come look at the dog that afternoon, I race like a lunatic out to a suburb I've never heard of.

The dog is beyond adorable. She jumps as high as a flea, is big on personality, and appears to be smiling all the time. She is a born kisser, a natural nuzzler.

And she barks.

I already know that I am going to say yes, but before I can reach for my checkbook, the breeder, all professionalism, brings out the puppy's AKC papers just to show me that her credentials are bona fide. She doesn't know poor old Lucy was a mutt; she doesn't know that it wouldn't matter to me if these AKC papers were counterfeit.

I know that I am going to name the puppy Charley Sloan, in honor of the character Bill created in *Shadow of a Doubt* and *Death Penalty*. But to be polite, I look at the papers anyway. Birth date: February 27; Bill's birthday is February 26.

Later that day, Jane stops by as she has been stopping by every Saturday since the Saturday Bill died, in memoriam, with her bunch of flowers and her heart the size of Texas.

Charley licks her face, nips at her ankles, runs around in puppy zooms, performing, in general, like the class clown.

"Oh, Ruth," says Jane, "she's just perfect. This one's a keeper, I just know it."

"Let's hope so," I reply. "Lately, my track record on keeping hasn't been too terrific."

We have made it to 1992.

New Year's Eve is a holiday neither Bill nor I especially care about. Mostly we have stayed home, snug and tucked away from the mayhem of the roads, content to watch the ball drop in Times Square from the comfort of wherever we were living, content to be happy, whole, and safe.

I remember the one year, though, that we opted for romance. Black floor-length dress and satin pumps for me, bare shoulders; best suit and shirt for him, holiday tie. Champagne on ice and lots of Frank Sinatra. Just the two of us, moving together on wall-to-wall carpeting, which, as you might imagine, is not the easiest feat to pull off when you're dancing.

But we did the fox-trot to the old tunes, especially to our signature song, "I'm Glad There Is You," to which we had also danced one night beneath the stars in Hawaii, the music emanating from a tinny radio in the house we had rented on the beach. Yes, it was corny, and yes, it was foolishly sentimental, but life is sometimes like that. Or, at least, it was.

This year, 1992, there is no thought of watching the ball

drop. December 1991 has been an exhausting month for Bill, and both of us are asleep well before midnight. Besides, the notion of wishing each other a Happy New Year is out of the question. It is seven months past the diagnosis, but neither of us mentions this. Neither of us notes, at least not out loud, that Bill has survived beyond the doctor's original prognosis.

In fact, he appears to rally during the month of January. He begins writing another Charley Sloan novel, he starts preparing the taxes to pass on to our accountant, he goes back to work, although his office has not scheduled him to hear any cases and although he does not put in a full day.

Because he is on so many medications, we have both decided that it would be best if I become the family driver, which, because Bill is not at all comfortable with my driving—and for good reason—has its humorous elements. Whereas he is a good driver, confident, sure, and verging on aggressive, I am just the opposite. The fact is I hate to drive, never needed to in New York, and I am uneasy behind the wheel. I hang in the slow lane, tenuous though steady, rarely moving into the middle lane to pass another car.

I am not secure in my new role. I am driving us to work almost every day and to the clinic at least once a week, and throughout every trip I can see that on the passenger side, Bill's right foot on the floorboard is working overtime.

He does not say a word, but you can cut the tension with a knife. It is more than just the fact that he is not crazy about the way I drive. That he has now been forced into the position of having his wife chauffeur him about is what is really getting to him. This unexpected circumstance is probably more humiliating to him than the time when he was autographing one of his books at a Kmart and the takers were so few that the store made him a blue-light special. It was a story he told on himself with glee, dining out on it, as he did, for years, embellishing it each time he told it, making it even more hilarious than it was the time before.

His book-signing days are over and he can no longer drive. As uncomfortable as my car is, low-slung and too small for him to get in and out of easily, he insists that I drive it instead of his.

"You're just a little bitty thing," he says, "you can hardly see over the dashboard in my car. It's much too big for you. Let's take yours." As he struggles into the car, he says the same thing every morning: "Don't forget to buckle up."

About using my car instead of his, he says very nearly the same words each day, and each day I try to tell him how senseless he is being. To no avail. Sick or not, he is still the most stubborn man I have ever met, but now I know that his stubbornness has taken on an edge.

I will do anything to please him, and as I acknowledge this, I try to remember if I felt that way before June 28. But, I realize, for the moment it is difficult for me to recall much of anything that took place before that date, and besides, what does it matter now?

Now I am taking care of a dying man. Now I will do anything he asks. Now I will shut my eyes tight and hope that my behavior, let us say the new me, does not seem wildly divergent from, let us say, the old me, the way I was before my husband became sick, when he was simply my husband and not a dying man.

On the road, I change my habits, becoming a regular Mario Andretti, driving in the fast lane, passing slowpokes at every opportunity. My hands are tight on the wheel, but I can see that my new aggressive stance has made Bill more relaxed in the passenger seat.

To make him laugh, I even adopt some of his habits. Like swearing at other drivers. Like talking to the ones with double-digit IQs as though they could hear you from one car to another.

To tell you the whole truth, I'm doing a pretty good imitation of Bill. "Come *on*," I mutter to a woman who's putting on her mascara in the rearview mirror and swerving from lane to lane. "Pretend that you have a real license. Make believe you didn't get it at Sears Roebuck." I turn to Bill and see that I have made him smile. If he is not happy, whole, and safe, I think, at least he is now more comfortable with my driving.

Two weeks of my chauffeurship pass before I notice what I should have seen right away.

Halfway into our trip to the clinic one day, I look over at Bill, just to see how he is doing.

He is not wearing his seat belt.

It is the first time I have ever seen him in a car without

one. My initial instinct is to tell him to buckle up, but I check myself quickly.

Knowing my husband as I do, I know that his not buckling the belt is intentional and not an oversight.

What could safety matter to him? He is on an ice floe, and no strip of nylon webbing will ever help him now.

I have taken to calling them They and Them.

Them and They comprise a loosely defined group of both things and people. The people: experts, writers, and such nonprofessionals as friends and acquaintances, sometimes family. The things: books and magazine pieces and newspaper articles. Often Their advice, solicited or unsolicited, is reasonable, valuable and important. Sometimes it is unwarranted, uncalled for, and—to me—unspeakably boorish.

"You know it takes a year for a widow to get over it," someone tells me. "On the other hand, with the loss of a child, it takes three."

Where do these projections come from?

Thinking about these seemingly arbitrary timetables, I become almost giddy, my mind performing pirouettes.

I imagine, according to these guidelines, this means that on April 25, 1993, I will spring back to life, embracing it with renewed vigor. Happy to be alive. Happy to be me. Eager to take on new challenges.

I recall Laurie telling me that it took her a year just to get beyond thinking how her mother, a cancer victim, looked at the end.

The twenty-fifth of April is three months from now. I hope that by then I will be more in control than I am now, that I will be better able to look forward rather than back, but I believe that I will have to undergo a lobotomy before I can say that I am "over it," whatever "over it" is supposed to mean.

I would like to be sanguine about the future, but I cannot forget what my mother told me many years ago. She had been named most optimistic girl in her high school graduating class. "Thanks for telling me," I'd said to her. "That explains, then, why you can be such an infuriating, mindless Pollyanna. Half of the time, you never touch base with reality."

"I suppose you're right," she'd countered. "So I guess I should tell you that my male counterpart, the kid who was also voted most optimistic, ultimately ended up in the booby hatch."

They have warned me that holidays and anniversaries and birthdays would be difficult. I have heard this from a dozen Theys, a dozen Thems. With an insufferable smugness, I thought that I would be immune. Armed with all these warnings, I reasoned, I wouldn't let it happen to me. I'm smarter than that, I'm better than that, I'm above all that.

Our wedding anniversary and Thanksgiving and Christmas, days spent without Bill, almost did me in. In this instance, They were right. Bill's birthday and the first-year anniversary of his death lie before me. Knowing what I now know, I am counting on being able to get through these days without collapsing like a hastily constructed Erector set.

One of the best ways to meet a new husband is to become involved in grief groups, I am told. Get it? All those widowers.

Knowing what I now know about mourning, it is impossible for me to imagine any widow, or widower, traipsing off to a grief group in search of a new companion, certainly not a husband or a wife. I am not fool enough to believe that men and women, like swans, mate for life, but to someone who is profoundly bereaved, the notion of being out there on the prowl is unthinkable.

"You know, a lot of people don't take this as hard as you're taking it," someone else says to me. I reply that I am certain this is true, but I cannot help wondering who those other people are and how they have managed to avoid falling into this sea of nothingness, how they have sidestepped this well of loneliness, how they have maneuvered through this tunnel with no light, either inside it or at the end of it.

I know that I will need to begin to let go of the past and look to the future. I know that there will come a time when letting go will seem more possible than it seems to me now, but for the moment I think it is a giant step for me to even acknowledge that there is a process known as letting go.

People have spoken to me about my lack of preparation, arguing that since I knew Bill was going to die, I should have been ready for it, less shocked, more serene. There is no such thing as preparation, I counter; while he was dying, it was all I could do to take care of him. Envisioning life without him was beyond my reach; you can't exactly liken the ten months of his illness to a fire drill and his death to the actual fire.

"I was not married to Bill," Jane tells me recently, "I was not family, either. But the vacuum for me is so much more enormous than I would have thought. In all the preparation I made, I was not ready for this. You just always expect people you love to be there."

"Did you ever stop and consider that maybe you loved him too much?" another person suggests. No, I have not considered that possibility, and had I considered it, what was I meant to do to stop loving him too much? How do you stop the sun from rising in the east?

"You mean you weren't working on your dependency problem, your overattachment to Bill, those six months you were in therapy?" a friend questions me. "What, for God's sake, were you doing that whole time?"

"Frankly," I reply, "what I was working on was trying to figure out a reason to get up in the morning."

It is amazing how you can lull yourself into a false sense of security.

During January, what with Bill's going back to work and with his writing the new book, I allow my thoughts of his impending death to diminish.

For his part, Bill appears to want everything to be as normal as possible. Certainly he is not the Bill Coughlin of a year ago, but after November and December and the fevers and the hospitalizations during those months, some of his strength is returning. He has long since stopped riding his Exercycle, but he can now shower without having to rest afterward. And walking up and down the stairs does not tire him as much.

It is amazing, too, how you will grab at any crumb that is thrown your way.

To say that he is chipper would not be a fair assessment, but he is more like himself, he is glad to see me back at the newspaper, he encourages me to leave the house more frequently than I have, assuring me that he is perfectly fine.

I do not remind him that he is not. Perfectly fine. It is such a joy to see him better—an odd choice of adjective, I realize—that I go along with whatever he says.

Go to Betsy's birthday party in Boston, he tells me. You've been friends for twenty years, you can't miss it, he says. After all, she's going to turn forty only once. At first I resist, but he is insistent.

"Toots," he says, "you can't be cooped up here forever. It's beginning to show on you, the strain, it's not good for your morale. And who's going to take care of me if you have a nervous breakdown?"

I work out a plan whereby I will be gone from him for a total of twenty-four hours, door to door, from our house to Logan Airport, to the party and the overnight stay with Betsy and Alan and their two daughters, Phoebe and Hilary, back to Logan, and then home.

With his customary generosity, Patrick quickly agrees to spend the day and night with his father, all of which goes off without a hitch.

When I come back, I tell Bill that while the party was swell and Betsy was glad to see me, it feels like I've been gone for a week; he says it seems to him like I've been away forever. "But look at you," he says, "you look better already. To tell you the whole truth, you look just splendid."

What I do not tell him is that after the party I have had a small crack-up in Betsy and Alan's guest room on the third floor of their house in Cambridge. Sobbing convulsively, I am unwittingly making enough noise to draw her from their bedroom. Attempting to console me, she can do nothing but put her arms around me as I rock back and forth and continue to weep.

Betsy, ever a woman of discretion and kindness, never mentions the incident again, and never do I tell my husband.

In an unusual piece of timing, there is, ten days later, another birthday party out of town, this one a surprise dinner to be given by Louise for her husband, Michael. It is being held in New York, and I can work out the same twenty-four-hour arrangement as I had worked out for the Betsy trip.

Once again, I need to be persuaded, and once again I let him do it.

"Ruth, it's Michael and Louise, they're two of our closest friends. You can't disappoint them. And remember, you had a great time at Betsy's. It did you good to get away."

But this time all is not smooth.

The night of the dinner party, January 30, I learn that my mother, who lives just outside of New York, has been rushed to the hospital. Four years earlier, she had undergone a life-threatening operation, and now she is suffering complications from that surgery. I will be in New York three days longer than planned, Patrick will be relieved by Maggie in staying at the house, and when I come back to Bill, I will be leaving my mother alone in a hospital where she will remain for the next five weeks.

One more time, I am forced to remember the conversation Bill and I had back in August. My father: gone. Lucy: gone. My mother: sick. My husband: sicker.

Will there ever be an end to this? It is a question I ask no one but myself.

And, of course, I already know the answer.

It is a harrowing month, the month of February. And while I do not know this for sure, I suspect that the ensuing days will be even more so.

Dr. Gordon has informed us that he is going to make an adjustment in Bill's chemotherapy treatment.

"The disease is clearly active," he tells us during a three-way telephone conversation. Bill and I both listen on separate extensions; I take the notes, using one of his yellow legal pads.

"We have slowed its progress," Dr. Gordon continues, "but it's still showing activity. We have to get it under control."

We are in separate rooms, Bill and I, side by side but separate, so I cannot see his expression, nor can I see what can be read in his eyes. On my end, I notice that my hand is trembling and that it is hard for me to hold the pen with which I am trying to jot down everything the doctor says.

In what sounds to me like an antidote to the gravity of what he has just told us, Dr. Gordon adds that there are other signs that indicate improvement. The liver cells, for instance, seem to have stabilized. He does not add anything more.

The next step that Dr. Gordon is about to outline is the one that my husband has been fearing all along. He has heard from friends and from friends of friends what it is like to be hospitalized for several days of chemotherapy. How gruesome the treatment is. How dreadful the aftereffects are. How it takes days after being discharged from the hospital to feel you are approaching anything close to normal.

We are told in specific detail what will take place during the five days that he is going to be treated, what to expect. There will be a combination of chemotherapy drugs administered intravenously over several hours' time, in addition to injections of platinum and caffeine, caffeine equivalent to fifteen to twenty cups of coffee. He will be given, by IV, something called Zofran, an anti-nausea drug that also acts as an amnesiac. His system will be bathed in IV fluids to protect his kidneys, which will be at risk of malfunctioning.

These drugs act in synergy, Dr. Gordon tells us, and they are, he adds, fairly well tolerated. A possible side effect is that Bill might develop some hearing problems whereby high-frequency sounds are lost. But we are not to worry: while these hearing problems are permanent in some cases, no one ever becomes fully deaf.

I think of bats.

I think of my husband's perfect imitation of the sounds that bats make, an imitation that has always provoked in me a fit of the giggles. Despite myself, despite the fact that I feel as if I am about to get sick, I smile at the memory of Bill being a bat.

We learn that once this treatment has been administered, sometimes a blood transfusion is necessary, but usually the transfusion doesn't take place until after two full cycles of the treatment.

"Do I have to go in right away?" Bill asks the doctor, who is more than well aware of how his patient feels about hospitals.

"Well, not this week. But I wouldn't wait three weeks," Dr. Gordon responds.

He ends our conversation in his usual cheerful manner, telling us to call him when we decide to come in so that he can alert the hospital. It is most definitely "we" this time; I will not let my husband go through this alone. I will live with him in the hospital, I will be at his side, I will sleep next to him in a fold-out chair, I will make certain that no one mistreats him.

I make a noisy display of gathering my notes together as I prepare to go into our bedroom where Bill is, and has been, during this conversation with the doctor. I have no idea what I am going to say, how I will look, how much of my own terror he will be able to detect.

"Well, it doesn't sound as though it'll be all that bad," I blurt out, knowing I am sounding like a moron. "And if it's true what he said about that Zofran stuff, then it looks as if you're going to forget or not even be aware of what's going on."

The more I say, the worse I sound. It occurs to me that I'm a little too old to be trying out for a cheerleader spot with the Dallas Cowboys, but I do not know any alternative. Between us we have set up a system of denial and deception, not by calculation, but simply because neither one of us knows how or when to start accepting the inevitable.

He looks at me steadily for just a few seconds, averts his eyes, glances out the window at his beloved trees, now barren and stark, and then his eyes seek out mine.

"Yeah, it won't be a walk in the park," he says, "that's for sure. But it's only five days. Hell, I used to tell my clients when they went to the slam they could do five years standing on their head, easy."

Both of us are getting very good at this game.

We are scheduled to go into the hospital on February 17, three days after Valentine's Day.

I have ordered a present for Bill—a leatherbound copy of *Shadow of a Doubt*—following a tradition I began when we first were married and as a wedding gift I presented him with a leatherbound copy of *No More Dreams,* one of his books on which I acted as editor. The book has not arrived from the bindery in time, but I am not overly upset. I can give it to him for his birthday on February 26, and surely I am not expecting a Valentine's Day present from him.

I am wrong.

From his trouser pocket he withdraws a small velvet box, navy blue. Inside are a pair of emerald-and-diamond earrings, demure and delicate. I am without words and close to bursting into tears, but I will not cry. He is so proud to have given me these earrings, the smile on his face is so utterly heartbreaking that I will not ruin this moment. When he tells me he's sorry he didn't get a chance to wrap the box, I am as near as I have ever been to going over the edge.

But so far, the game of charades we have tacitly chosen to

play, the one that disallows us from showing or saying what we feel about this catastrophe, seems to be working well, and I do not want to tip the balance.

The treatment at the hospital is no worse and no better than what we had expected: it is simply a nightmare. Bill is knocked out most of the time, but in those rare moments when he is awake, he is dry-heaving into a plastic bowl, his poor face screwed up, pathetically contorted. I am helpless. All I can do is hold the bowl; all I can do is lay my hand on his sad, shuddering back; all I can do is be there, wiping his mouth with a tissue, stroking his head, caressing his hand.

When he is heavily medicated and down for the count, I am relieved. I want them to give him even more drugs so that he doesn't know how awful this is, this darkened room, the machines murmuring, the almost silent drip of the IVs as the fluids seep slowly into his body, the eerie, surreal feel to what is happening to him and around him.

I read voraciously, two books a day, by the light of the lamp next to my fold-out bed. I cannot tell you what I read during those five days. I complete the crossword puzzles from three daily newspapers. Bill is so quiet it is scary, his breathing so soft and shallow that I constantly check to see if his chest is moving.

But I know that he is not dead, he is just dead to the world, a world which I now accept, as Jane has pointed out, is a cruel and unforgiving place.

I wander the halls in the hours past midnight, barefoot because I have forgotten to bring slippers. I call my mother in her hospital room every day, I talk to friends all across the country. As my husband sleeps a dreamless sleep, I am connected by pay phone to people on the outside, an environment foreign and remote, a place where Bill and I once used to live.

I make friends with the nurses, these remarkable women who are devoted to the care of the terminally ill. And make no mistake, 4 Yellow Center, where my husband is, is the cancer ward. There is Linda and Johnnie and Pam and Gwen. There is J.T. and Laura and Diane and Mary. There is Stephanie and Angie and Annette.

I proudly show them photographs of Bill, the before pictures; I give them copies of his books. I imagine that I am so overbearingly protective of him that at times they would like me just to go home, but I don't care. I won't go home.

There are the memorial plaques on the wall by the nurses' station, gifts of gratitude from the wives, the husbands, the families, the survivors. There are cards and letters and flowers and candy, displayed with pride by the nursing staff.

I find myself drawn to these cards and letters of appreciation, reading every one of them, even as I know what each one means: someone had to die before one of these notes was written. Someone did not walk out of 4 Yellow Center alive.

I ask Linda how she does it. How can she bear witness to this kind of suffering, day after day, week after week? Her answer is simple: she does it, she says, because if for one single moment she can make a dying patient more comfortable, she has then met her calling. She has accomplished what she has set out to do.

I think of my husband, two doors down, as still as water in a pond. While he has accomplished a great deal, it is not all that he had set out to do, and now, immobilized and impotent, the most he can do is receive the fluids that the medical profession hopes will extend his life. Extend it. Not save it.

They release him on February 22, and he enters our house as though he had been imprisoned in solitary confinement for ten years on a desert island.

It has been a dreadful time, he is depleted and worn down, but he is so happy to be home that his appreciation is contagious.

In time for his birthday, the leatherbound book arrives. Shakily, I inscribe it, knowing that inscribe it I must, just as I have inscribed his previous novels, rich in their green leather casings, lined up in a row on one shelf of a living-room bookcase: "For my one and only Will—The best for the best. No one even comes close. I love you."

Scott and Margaret and their son, the incomparable Michael, stop by for a visit, and Bill pays them the ultimate compliment when he tells me after they leave that these young people remind him of his parents.

As February moves into March, he is eating less and growing more lethargic. March will bring the return of Kathleen from San Diego, and that of Dennis and his family from Oklahoma. It will see me flying to New Jersey to spring my mother from the hospital, while Billy and Patrick take care of their father.

It will see the opening of Patrick's new jewelry store, an opening that Bill refuses to miss. He is wan and weak, but there is no stopping him from our driving the more than forty miles to St. Clair to congratulate Patrick. This time, he takes the wheel himself, in what I know is a symbolic gesture.

March will see visits by Jack and Marge and Jane and Larry and the Coughlin children and grandchildren.

And it will see, on March 13, the retirement of William J. Coughlin, a man who vowed repeatedly that he would never retire, would never relinquish either of his professions; his appointment to the federal bench was a lifetime appointment, and his dedication to the writing of his books was a self-imposed lifetime appointment as well.

He would, he told me, never lie fallow, never be inactive, never not contribute.

As I look back now—even though I know that the disease had begun to take over, even though I know that his will and his body had used every remaining scrap of strength to fight the good fight—I think that the day his retirement became official was the day that his final descent began.

Somehow, I missed menopause.

I suppose it began during my husband's illness, but I didn't take much notice.

Sure, it seemed as if I was overly warm at times, flushing from my toes to the top of my head. Guess this is what they call hot flashes, I would say to myself, and then I would say, hey, Bill, what do you know? Looks like I'm going through menopause.

You would be guessing right if you wagered that he urged me to see my gynecologist. Pressed me, would be more accurate, and therefore I did.

The wait was so long, I left. I had no time to be sitting in a doctor's office, no patience, either. As I stormed out of the waiting room, it occurred to me that menopause was no big deal. Stack your basic menopause against your basic terminal cancer, and there would be no contest.

After he died, the flashes, if that was in fact what they were, got worse. Bigger. More intense. Much more frequent. At night I'd be bathed in sweat, my legs slippery, slithering off the bed as I rushed to throw open the windows.

But then I remembered reading somewhere that anxiety attacks, or worse, panic attacks, could produce the exact same effect. There was no question in my mind that I was panicky, that lurid dreams awakened me in the middle of the night, that a good deal of the time I felt as though an elephant were sitting on my chest.

Just panic, not menopause, I told myself. No big deal.

As the months wore on, these nighttime sweats grew more exaggerated, and I realized, too, that not only had I missed seeing my gynecologist, I had also forgotten the date of my last mammogram. It was probably years ago. Given the manner in which my husband had just died, probably not such a good idea.

The mammogram appointment goes off smoothly; I do not give it a second thought. The results will be back in about a week, and I do not even make a note to remind myself to call the doctor's office. This is certainly not my first mammogram, and there has never before been a problem.

Clean slate. Easy breezy. Nothing to worry about.

The phone call comes on a Wednesday morning, early.

There is, Dr. Butler tells me, something in my left breast. It is small, he says, but it is, nonetheless, there. He assures me that more than likely it is just a benign cyst, but I am remembering May 1991 when a group of doctors told my husband and me that what appeared to be on his liver was just some fatty tissue.

He did not live to see May 1992.

He would like me to see Dr. Donald J. Weaver for a consultation. I know this doctor; he is a likable and competent man who performed two procedures on my husband, and as I remember him, he is a surgeon.

"What are you doing sending me to a cutter?" I ask Dr. Butler, hysteria in my voice. I am overreacting, I know, but I cannot help it.

Dr. Weaver, I am told, is a nationally known breast specialist, and yes, he is also a surgeon. Arrangements will be made for me to see him in a couple of weeks.

"Two weeks?" I fairly shout. "You expect that after having watched my husband die from cancer I'm going to wait around for two weeks to find out if this thing is malignant or not?"

The appointment is moved up by ten days, and then I am left, except for Charley, alone in the house. My tough-guy telephone talk is gone, and it is me, just me. And a possibly malignant tumor in my left breast.

I need to talk to Bill. I need to have him stand by me as I begin to shake uncontrollably, and as my sobs turn into shrieks. I need for him to comfort me, to rub my back, to take me to the doctor. I need everything about him, his strength, his courage, his dignity.

As I think this, a ghostly calm comes over me.

Remember June 28, 1991, I remind myself. He did not react the way you are reacting right now, and you have been informed only that there is a cyst in your left breast.

No one has told you that you have terminal cancer. No one has even suggested it. Take charge, be big, not small. Grow up, accept whatever is handed to you.

This calm lasts for maybe thirty minutes, and then I turn demented again. Now I am convinced that if I have cancer, it is probably just as well. A life without Bill is no life at all, I tell myself, so this is clearly meant to be.

I am trying to find some smooth air, but it does not seem likely. Somewhere between hoping I have cancer, a truly insane thought, and believing that a life without Bill is not worth living, a possibly insane thought, there has to be a middle ground.

Dr. Weaver's office is in the same building as the oncology clinic where I have not been for seven months, except that his offices are on a different floor. I can drive there blindfolded, my hands off the wheel. It is home ground now; it is, in its own aberrant way, terra firma.

The same homeless people whose cardboard placards say they will work for food are on the streets. They are even manning the exact same corners. The same man is in charge of valet parking. The same attendant is in the building's lobby.

It is as though nothing has changed, but of course everything has. I used to have Bill, and now I do not. I used to have a life, and now I do not. I can do nothing about the former, but there must be something I can do about the latter.

The design of the building is such that each floor is a

replica of the others. Before going to see Dr. Weaver, I press the elevator for the oncology clinic, knowing that I have to do this. I must go back before I can go forward.

As I walk down the hallway to the reception area, I think that I feel a swirl of cold air surround me, but I know of course that to think this is absurd.

And then I am upon it, the room where we sat week after week. The sign-in desk where I signed him in; the cashier's office where I paid the bills. The furniture has not changed but the plants look droopy, old, neglected.

I am Emily Webb in Grover's Corners. I see Bill in the chair he always chose to sit in, I see him as he takes off his coat and scarf and his gloves. I see us sitting side by side, our arms touching. I see myself nodding off, my head falling onto his shoulder. I see us moving into a back cubicle where brilliantly colored poisons will be dripped into his body.

I have seen enough.

In Dr. Weaver's office, I learn that the cyst is just that: a cyst. It is not malignant, I do not have cancer, and it is good to see Dr. Weaver, always a comforting presence, again.

As I get ready to leave, he asks how I am doing. "Not bad," I say, the usual. But because he was, briefly, one of Bill's doctors, this time I add, "None of this is easy."

"You know, your husband was a remarkable man," he says.

"Yes, I know that," I respond. "Thank you," I add, as though in any way I were responsible for how remarkable he was.

"You know how much he affected everyone he met, don't you?" he asks.

"Yes, I do know that," I reply, dropping the thank you.

"You must be so . . ." he pauses for more than a few seconds, obviously looking for the right word, "I mean, you must be so . . ."—he pauses again—"so alone."

It is the first time someone other than I has actually uttered the word with such stunning clarity and simplicity, and at first it is astonishing to hear it.

"Yes, I am," I say. "I am alone."

At the end of March, Bill is back in the hospital for ten days, and I live with him there. There is another cycle of chemotherapy, but during these ten days his heart rate reaches unnatural highs, and, because of this, there are new drugs added to his daily regimen.

But he is, incredibly enough, still cheerful.

On March 30, for the first time in our life together, he stays awake with me to watch the Academy Awards to the very end. In years past, he'd go to sleep before the big awards were announced, leaving me to report to him first thing in the morning who won. His staying up with me this year, in a hospital room and not in our own house, I see as a sign. He knows this is the last one.

We come back home on April 2, and the next day a visiting nurse from the Michigan Cancer Society is sent to see Bill. She is a charming and attractive woman, and in the outrageous-flirt category she has met her match. I marvel as I see this interchange, one charmer to another, take place before me. I cannot believe this, I think to myself, he never changes.

A month at the most is what the nurse tells me when we both go downstairs after she has finished with Bill.

On the seventh of April, I call an ambulance to take him back to the hospital for a blood transfusion. An ambulance, his second biggest phobia.

I have never had to call for an ambulance before in my life, nor has Bill ever had occasion to be in one. The attendants, a young woman and a young man, are no-nonsense and not especially comforting; the one-way, mirrored sunglasses he is wearing and never takes off go a long way toward adding to this sinister scene. And maybe, just maybe, she could stop chewing that damn gum.

As they begin to strap Bill onto the stretcher, I recall the first time I ever saw him in a wheelchair. That was bad enough; this is almost too much to bear.

In my youth, I have been part of crews helping friends move from place to place, so even I know that the strongest person should be at the foot of an object that is being brought down a flight of stairs. This is no object, this is my husband, and for a reason that will never be known, the young woman—shorter than I, and I am very short—takes the position at the bottom of the stretcher, and the young man—at least six-feet-four and burly—takes the top, his mirrored sunglasses firmly in place.

Halfway down the steps, Bill begins to slide off the stretcher, but miraculously this gruesome twosome somehow doesn't let it happen. Once outside, they do not let me ride in the back with him. Against regulations, they tell me. State law. I have never heard of this state law, but then again

I have never been in an ambulance before. I am furious, but this is hardly the time for me to show my fury.

It is an outpatient, daylong procedure, this blood transfusion, the second one he has had. It is very tedious and Bill is short on patience. But we spend the day together, watching a stranger's dark, thick blood being infused into his body, chatting about nothing in particular.

As I am fluffing up a pillow for him, he takes hold of my wrist and quietly says, "You know, you never know what you have until you're about to lose it."

He is more tired than he has ever been, and when some of the children and I bring him back home—he refuses the hospital's offer of an ambulance—he immediately goes to bed, a bed he will never leave again.

That afternoon I need to make a drugstore run, and before I do, Bill asks me if I could do something for him. Because we knew that the cancer had metastasized to the liver, the primary site never to be discovered, Bill has not had a single drink for ten months. Now he wonders if I might pick up some bourbon for him and maybe a little soda to mix it with.

"No problem," I say. "I'll buy a fifth."

"Let's not be that optimistic," Bill responds. "A pint should do it."

As this exchange takes place, I can feel my heart plummeting to my shoes. He's having a drink because he knows he's getting close to the end. It doesn't matter to him anymore that the bourbon will go straight to his liver. I am sure about what he is thinking: he is thinking, what difference could it possibly make now? I am also aware that he knows I know, but, as has become our custom, neither of us openly acknowledges this.

I mix the bourbon and soda when I come back. Because it has become difficult for Bill to swallow, I slip a straw into the glass and carry it upstairs.

"One bourbon and soda coming right up," I lamely chirp, sounding like a bird with a broken wing. I am relieved to see that he is reading and listening to his radio, alert and, to my eye, oddly chipper.

He takes one sip through the straw, and then places the drink on the table beside him, a small, lingering smile on his lips, mischief in his eyes.

"Somebody around here," he says, now laughing, "is out of practice. I never would have believed you'd forget how to mix a good drink."

Another sip. Ten minutes go by, and he is fast asleep.

Hours later, I will remove the drink, its contents once rich and dark and amber now pale and diluted, the ice cubes long gone, the straw leaning up against the side of the glass, a white ring of water indelibly stamped on the table.

The house is filled with people this month of April. Bill's children who are single, his sons and their wives and their children, my friends, his friends, our friends. We can set our clocks by Jane, who arrives every evening at seven o'clock. Day and night we sit in the living room, one of us running upstairs every few minutes to check on Bill, who is now sleeping most of the time.

We are sitting shivah in reverse. We are mourning him as his life begins to draw slowly to a close, about twenty years too soon. We are waiting for him to die

One night there is a terrible storm, the earsplitting thunder shaking the windows of the house. "If this doesn't wake him up," someone says, "nothing will." From upstairs, I hear him call my name. He is wide awake. "Are you okay?" I ask as I rush into the bedroom. "Some storm, huh?" he says. "Why don't you lie down next to me and I'll take care of you."

Because he is on morphine, and liquid Thorazine and Ativan, he is in and out of reality, dreamy and not like himself one minute, perfectly lucid and very much like himself the next. But mostly he sleeps.

"You're the kind of girl they make diamonds for," he says to me one morning, his lips forming a sweet, far-away smile. "Will you just stop talking?" he snaps at me another day, although I do not remember talking too much. One night, I wake with a start. Bill is sitting up on the side of the bed; I cannot imagine how he has been able to do this without help. "Tootsie?" he whispers. "Are they coming to shoot me now?"

A visiting nurse, because it is part of her job, decides to test him with the usual questions. Who is the president? What day is it? How old are you? Because I am never out of the room when either a doctor or a nurse is with him, I am there to witness what I perceive to be this brutally degrading questioning. I am quick to action, hastily making a sign on a yellow legal pad. In huge block letters I write NO MORE QUESTIONS and hold it up to her in a way that she can see it and he cannot.

I later tell the nurse I know what she is doing and why she is doing it, but we both know that he is dying and there is no point in putting him through these tests. I tell her if she had known him before he got sick she would be amazed at how smart he was, how handsome he was, how funny he was. I am babbling, I know, and she is kind enough not to stop me.

Another nurse who arrives to bathe him somehow has decided that he cannot hear her. It is an arduous task bathing him in bed, and as I help with the job, I don't know how to ask her to lower her voice without sounding imperious. She is talking to him as though he were two years old and she is shouting at the top of her lungs.

"I'm not deaf, dear," Bill gently tells her. "I can hear you just fine."

As the days wear on, the circumstances turn more surreal. To see him this way, drugged, unable to get out of bed, barely able to sit up, is torture. The single consolation is that he is so heavily medicated that he is not in pain. At least that is what I tell myself.

People come and go throughout the days and nights, bringing food and drink and cigarettes and endless supplies of support. I will not leave the house. What if he dies while I'm gone? One afternoon someone convinces me to get out for just a little while, and I agree. I go to the supermarket and am attacked by a panic so acute that I turn around and come home almost immediately.

On Friday, April 24, he has deteriorated to such a degree that I know I have to ask Dr. Gordon to come to the house. We have been in touch by telephone throughout the whole month; he has been in contact with all the Michigan Cancer Foundation nurses who have been stopping by, but the last time the doctor actually saw Bill was in the hospital on April 7, the day of the transfusion.

He arrives Friday evening; there are, as there have been since April 7, at least a dozen people in the living room. He knows how grave the situation is, but I warn him before we go upstairs that Bill's condition is bad, very bad. I tell him that the nurse who had seen him earlier in the day suggested that he would not live through the weekend. As I tell him these things, I realize how unnecessary my comment is: he is an oncologist, he has seen dying people many times before, he has more experience in this than I do.

Bill is glad to see him, even asks him how he's doing. He is partly dozing, partly awake, but not unconscious; and the doctor treats his patient as he has for the past ten months— with respect and admiration and enormous compassion.

That night Dr. Gordon sits with me at the kitchen table for more than two hours, gabbing, telling stories, making me laugh. He talks to the others who come in and out of the kitchen to replenish various supplies. While I am tremendously grateful to him for having come to see Bill, while I am also appreciative for his spending all this time at our house, I can't help but wonder why, in fact, he is spending all this time.

And then I get it.

This is his farewell, this is his own grieving process. In his own way, he is saying good-bye to his patient, the man he has treated and gotten to know well during the past ten months. He knows, although he won't actually say it, that this is the last time he will see Bill alive. For him, this is closure.

I know that Saturday, April 25, 1992 will be the last day of my husband's life.

I know this as I wake up in the morning, as I touch his body while he is sleeping next to mine.

I shower, I get dressed, I know this is the day.

Starting in the early morning, the children and I take turns sitting in a chair drawn close to the bed. Fifteen-minute vigils, like a watch at sea.

Toward the end, all of us gather in the room together, each of us saying good-bye in our own way. Bill is in and out of consciousness, his eyes closed, his breathing alternating between great heaving gasps and small almost undetectable sighs.

He cannot speak, he is drowning in his own fluids, but he will not let go.

For two hours and six minutes we watch him hold on, we watch him struggle. When he chokes out two small words—*help me*—there is nothing we can do. We are helpless, people without power; there is nothing we can do but tell him that we love him.

It is the agony of the Cross.

"Billy, Billy," I whisper in his ear at five-minute intervals, "please, please, please, baby, please just let go. You don't have to fight anymore. You can give it up."

Maggie, who has been monitoring his blood pressure, looks up and gives us the warning. "Okay, this is it," she says.

I am kneeling on the floor next to the bed, holding his hand. I am aware that the room is filled with the sounds of keening, and there is a curious ringing in my ears.

My husband's eyes fly open. Wide. In shock, I must imagine. In horror, I must imagine. Or, maybe, in fear.

They are bluer than I have ever seen them before.

His hand drops from mine.

His eyes, unseeing, remain open.

His beautiful face begins to turn blue.

"Please," I sob, my body shaking. "Please. Somebody please close his eyes."

It is finished.

I call the cops. I call the doctor. I call the undertakers. I call my mother. I call Jane, hating to leave a message on her machine, but knowing that I must and knowing that I will not be able to get through this day without her and Larry.

The only preparation I have made for this is to have put together a list of thirty or so people who need to be told that Bill is dead. Scott, who has been in the house the whole time, takes the list out of my hands. Tough, unflappable street reporter that he is, he begins methodically making the calls. Laura, who had stopped by to visit earlier in the day and had left to see our friend Anne Marie, arrives just as the police pull up.

The two cops make a strange couple, the older one is pure business; he has no doubt been in this situation a thousand times before. The rookie is wandering through the house making comments about the wood paneling in one room, the tile in another. Why is the kid a cop? I think to myself. He should have been Mario Buatta.

Billy and Patrick and Dennis help me choose the suit, the tie, the suspenders, the shirt, the silk pocket square. I make sure to slip a cigar and a stick of gum, spearmint, in my husband's jacket pocket.

When the hearse pulls up, I can feel my knees beginning to buckle. Two undertakers and a stretcher. I lead them to Bill.

As I am walking back downstairs, I can hear them close the bedroom door.

What seems like hours later but isn't, I hear the pop of the door being opened.

This is it, I say to myself. A black body bag. Zipped. My husband in it. They are bringing him down.

I slowly walk to the staircase as I sense people forming in line in back of me. I cannot tell you how many people. There is a hushed silence. We are paying homage. No one moves, no one makes a sound. It is as quiet as a cathedral.

As I look to the top of the stairs, I see one undertaker's back. I see his black shoe touch the first step, then the second, and then the third. Behind me, I hear the sound of a muffled cry.

I am riveted. I have turned to stone.

They are on the fourth step.

I can see the foot of the bag.

"If you drop him," I say, "I will fucking kill you."

I am sleeping in our bed.

"Which side?" the bereavement counselor asks me.

"Bill's, of course," I answer. "I like it there." Charley sleeps on the pillow that used to be mine.

Ten months later, the nightmares, both waking and sleeping, occur less frequently. I do not think as often about how I stood in the doorway and waved good-bye as the hearse pulled away from the house.

I am getting better at the pronouns. I can now say "I" with more ease. I can get through whole days without crying.

I can talk to people about the funeral, listen to Laura when she tells me that of course Bill didn't look like Bill but that after standing around with him in the viewing room for two days, she got to like having him in the room. "My life changed when Bill died," she tells me. "I feel more connected to what it means to die. I have a more real sense now of how finite life is."

I would be lying if I said that I do not reread some of the

letters that people sent to me. I do. "Bill was one of the finest people I've ever met," writes Betsy. "He reminded me of the best qualities of my father: brains, talent, humor, and beneath it all, profound kindness."

While my first instinct was to sell the house, I am staying. At least for now. I try to concentrate on the good memories here, not the bad.

Whole conversations take place in which I do not mention Bill's name. I imagine it is less fraught with pain to talk to me now than it was ten months ago.

These days I am better able to remember Bill as he was before he got sick rather than after. I have found a video tape of a television interview he once did, but I know that I am not yet ready to play it. I know that I need to move forward, not backward, but I also know that someday in the future I will slip the tape into the VCR and be happy to see him again.

I have started to go through his desk. I can now do this for more than five minutes at a time. I have found a cassette tape, audio notes Bill made to himself while writing one of his novels. I have played it just once, both startled and frightened at first to hear the sound of his voice. By the end of the tape, I found it comforting. I will not throw out the cassette.

I have found unused cotton balls, some loose change, a few photographs of me, correspondence that goes back to the 1950s, old magazines, and a magnifying glass.

Way at the back of the middle drawer, I have found a tiny

gold boxing glove, a memento from his youth and his days in the ring. I have never before seen this glove. On it is engraved WILLIAM J. COUGHLIN, CHAMP.

I have accepted the fact that my husband is dead, but I know, too, that he will never leave me and I will never be without him. I know that I can let go and continue on to the next phase of my life without giving him up.

The lyrics of our song run through my mind less frequently, but it is our song and always has been. And so it will remain:

> In this world of ordinary people, extraordinary
> people, I'm glad there is you.
> In this world of overrated pleasures, of under-
> rated treasures, I'm glad there is you.
> In this world where many, many play at love
> And hardly any stay in love
> I'm glad there is you
> More than ever, I'm glad there is you.

Is you.
Was you.
Is you.

Epilogue

What follows is the eulogy I wrote during the morning of the first day of Bill's wake. I was hoping to read it myself, but it quickly became apparent that I would be incapable of doing so. Coming to the rescue as he has dozens of times in the past, our great friend Michael Dorris, who had traveled on four airplanes to be present at the funeral, delivered me from my predicament and managed, quite remarkably, to read the letter with elegance and grace. I do not know how he did it. But I do know that both Michael and Bill played to a packed house.

April 25th, 1992

Dearest Billy,

Since how we met was by mail, and what wonderful letters they were, it seems only appropriate to me that I write you this one last letter.

In the beginning, you were in Detroit, a place where I had never been, I was in New York, and I asked you if Detroit had an airport. Since then, lots of things have changed. For instance, I now know that Detroit has an airport.

But here are some of the other things I now know.

I know that in the all-too-short time we had together that you were my hero.

I know that until I met you I knew nothing about brilliance and dignity and courage and the generosity of spirit.

I know that I will never again meet a man who three days before he died told me that I'm the kind of girl they make diamonds for.

It is true that we didn't agree on everything. You believed in the right to bear arms, while I believed that every firearm in the world should be destroyed. I thought going to the movies wasn't such a bad idea, and you always wanted to wait for the video.

In the end, though, because we had each other, it was all small potatoes.

And because we shared an appreciation for the written word, I thought you would like to hear this passage from one of our all-time favorite writers.

It's from an essay called "John Wayne: A Love Song," and I don't even need to tell you who wrote it:

"We went three and four afternoons a week, sat on folding chairs in the darkened Quonset hut which served as a theater, and it was there, that summer of 1943 while the hot wind blew outside, that I first saw John Wayne. Saw the walk, heard the voice. Heard him tell the girl in a picture called *War of the Wildcats* that he would build her a house 'at the bend in the river where the cottonwoods grow.' As it happened I did not grow up to be the kind of woman who is the heroine of a Western, and although the men I have known have had many virtues and have taken me to live in many places I have come to love, they have never been John Wayne, and they have never taken me to that bend in the river where the cottonwoods grow."

So, Billy, here is the big difference between me and Joan Didion: for nine years, you have taken me to that bend in the river where the cottonwoods grow. For nine years, you gave me the gift of you.

I don't even know how to begin to thank you, and I don't even know how to begin to tell you how sorry I am that this vicious and grotesque killer got you. While the day you died was not a perfect day for bananafish, it was, however, the day that finally took you out of your pain, for which I am grateful.

Rest in peace, pal.

Write me a letter when you think of it.

Acknowledgments

The list seems endless, but a list there must be, for without these people there would have been no book.

I would like to offer my gratitude to the following:

To the Coughlin children—Margaret, William, Susan, Dennis, Patrick, and Kathleen. Thank you for lending me your father.

To my mother, Sonia Pollack, and my brother, Michael J. Pollard. Thank you for being my family.

To Dr. Craig J. Gordon, whose compassion and zeal know no bounds; and to Fayette Loria and David R. Hough for helping me make it through the night.

To Robert H. Giles, Julia S. Heaberlin, Martin A. Fischhoff, and Pam Shermeyer of *The Detroit News:* Thank you for your kindness during the ten months of my husband's illness.

To my friends and to my husband's friends, our friends, for their steadfast, and, in some cases, superhuman support: John and Maureen Barron; Wes Bausmith; Kitty Benedict; Laura Berman (thank you for being my check on reality and for catching me every time I fell) and Chris Norris; Anne

Marie Biondo; George Bulanda; Lynn Coughlin; Sandra DeVito; Michael Dorris and Louise Erdrich; Roy Figurski; Michael S. Green; Betsy Groban and Alan B. Fischer; Julie Hinds; Reed Johnson and Marla Dickerson; Kathy Kaczanowski; Marney Rich Keenan; Tim Kiska; Kelly Kolhagen; Lesley Krauss; Joanna Krotz and Wayne Kuhn; Scott, Margaret, and Michael Martelle; Michael McWilliams; Jack and Marge Mease; Ivy Millerand; Alicia and David Nordquist; the Hon. Thomas J. O'Dowd; Allen H. Peacock; Charles E. Spicer; Susan Stark.

To Jane Rayburn and Larry McDaniel, whose largesse cannot be measured and whose love will never be forgotten.

To Charles Rembar, my agent, whose sense and sensibilities continue to stay the course.

To Charley Sloan, both of them.

To the artistry of a peerless fleet of Random House professionals—Enrica Gadler, Jean-Isabel McNutt, Robbin Schiff, Peter Vertes, Carol Schneider—and, most especially, to my editor and longtime friend, Ann Godoff, the wind beneath my wings.

ABOUT THE AUTHOR

RUTH COUGHLIN is an award-winning feature writer; she has been the book editor for *The Detroit News* since 1985. Before moving to Detroit in 1983, she worked in New York publishing. She is a past board member of the National Book Critics Circle, having served as vice president for publications for three years. She lives in Grosse Pointe, Michigan.

ABOUT THE TYPE

This book was set in Bembo, a typeface based on an old-style Roman face that was used for Cardinal Bembo's tract *De Aetna* in 1495. Bembo was cut by Francisco Griffo in the early sixteenth century. The Lanston Monotype Machine Company of Philadelphia brought the well-proportioned letter forms of Bembo to the United States in the 1930's.